FOR THE LOVE OF BUCKWHEAT

FROM APPETIZER TO DESSERT

MARIA DEPENWEILLER

For the Love of Buckwheat
Copyright © 2020 by Maria Depenweiller

Photography images belongs to Maria Depenweiller

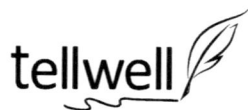

tellwell

Tellwell Talent
www.tellwell.ca

ISBN
978-0-2288-2850-1 (Hardcover)
978-0-2288-2849-5 (Paperback)

Getting to know the grain

Whole grains are a gold mine of useful nutrients and a cornerstone of any traditional diet. Plain grains, noodles, flo
there is an endless variety of products made with various grains that are eaten all over the world. Yet some grain
much more well-known than others, depending on the geographical region. I would like to introduce you to buckw
— the wonder grain of cold climate regions. Its popularity spans through France, Eastern Europe and the northern c
of Japan. I am sure it will impress you with the versatility and simplicity of the dishes. But before we start cooking, let'
to know buckwheat a bit closer.

Buckwheat is not a cereal

Buckwheat (*Fagopyrum esculentum*) is a sturdy, undemanding plant that is related to sorrel and dock. It is a vigc
grower, allowing for more than one crop per year. The virtue of buckwheat is that it thrives in poor soil, does not rec
intricate maintenance and has a short growing season, making it a perfect fit for regions with cold climates, poor soil
short summers. Seeds have a pyramidal shape and, according to the *Oxford Companion to Food*, were named beco
of their resemblance to beechnuts. The name buckwheat was most likely derived from Dutch — bockweit, mea
beechwheat. Buckwheat's origins can be traced back to Manchuria and Siberia where it was cultivated as early as
BC according to the *Cambridge World History of Food*. By the fourteenth and fifteenth centuries buckwheat had reac
Europe, and then in the seventeenth century the Dutch colonists brought it to the New World.

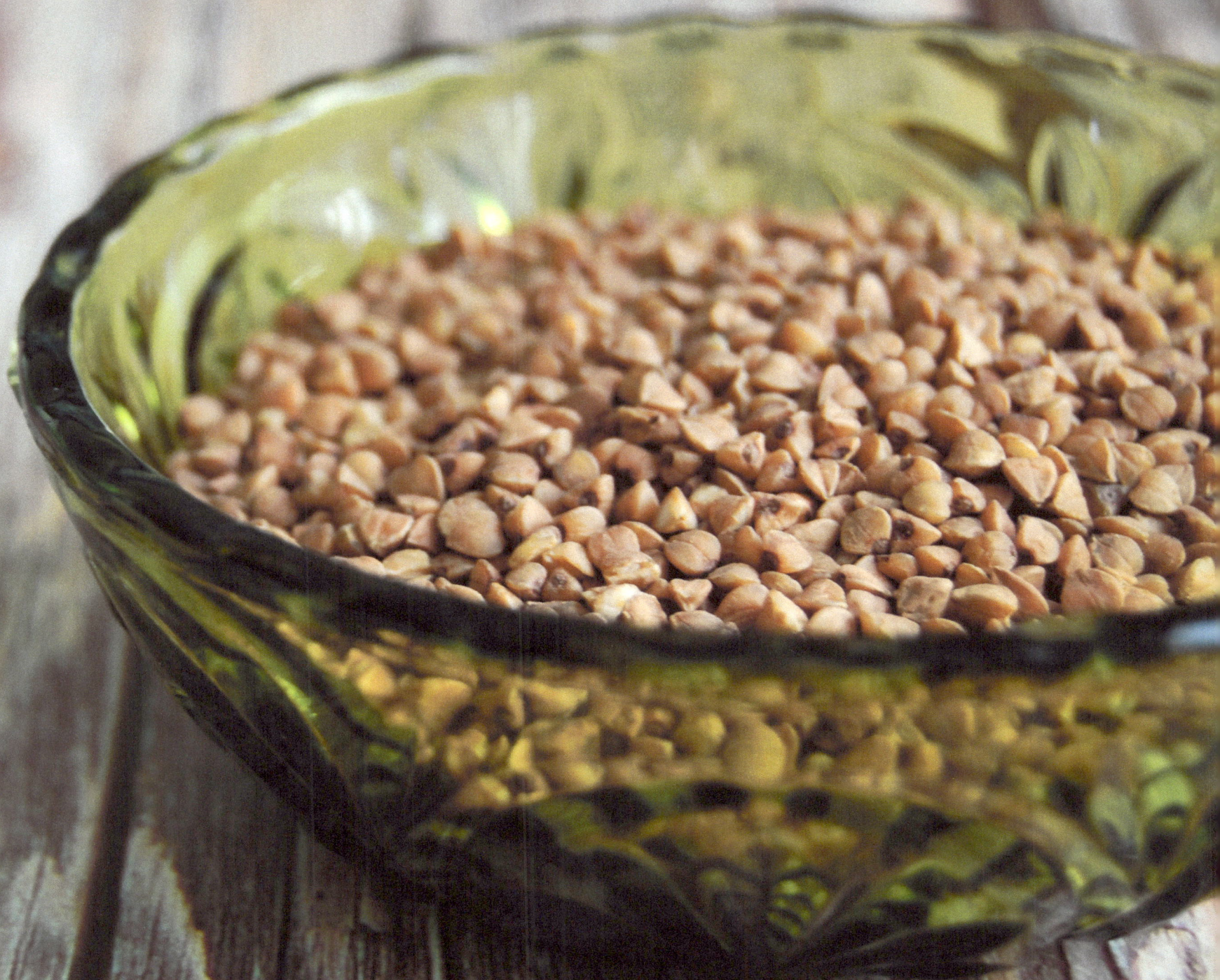

Packed with nutrition

Buckwheat grains are an excellent source of protein, containing all nine essential amino acids. Dietary fiber contain buckwheat grains is beneficial to the healthy function of the digestive tract. The low glycemic index of buckwhea its slow absorption rate makes it useful in controlling blood sugar levels, and its slow absorption rate means an impr feeling of satiety after a meal. Buckwheat is loaded with such important microelements as magnesium, phospho potassium, selenium, thiamin, riboflavin, vitamin K, rutin, folate and niacin. Together they help improve heart health, t health and they strengthen the immune system. As buckwheat is not related to wheat it is naturally gluten free a suitable for people who are allergic to wheat or have a gluten intolerance.

Bees love it too

Buckwheat is a great honey plant. It gives rich dark brown honey with very strong flavour. Situating bee hives or perimeter of the buckwheat field is an ancient natural way of increasing the harvest of the buckwheat because the p require pollination by bees for proper formation of the seed pods.

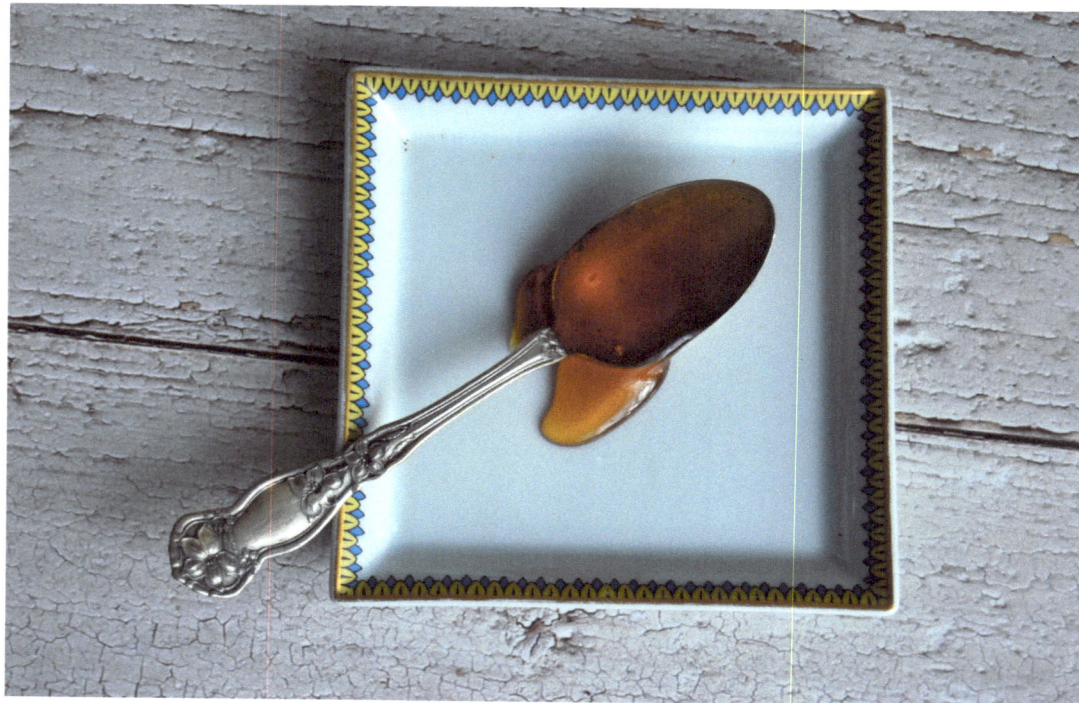

The entire plant is useful. Buckwheat seeds are eaten either roasted or cooked and are used to make flour. Buckwheat hulls, left from ripened seeds, are used to fill pillows and the green part of the buckwheat plant is an excellent forage for domestic animals. All in all, buckwheat creates zero waste and is beneficial to the environment.

I was born in a region where buckwheat was an important staple food and every member of our family had a preferred dish containing buckwheat. In a way, it was a comfort food either as a warm and welcoming breakfast porridge or a hearty stew on a frosty winter evening. In my mind buckwheat was a synonym of comfort and coziness.

Over the years I have discovered many new and wonderful recipes that use buckwheat in the form of grains or flour, and I would like to share my love for this wonderful plant with you, dear reader. I hope you will find your new favourite comfort food in this book.

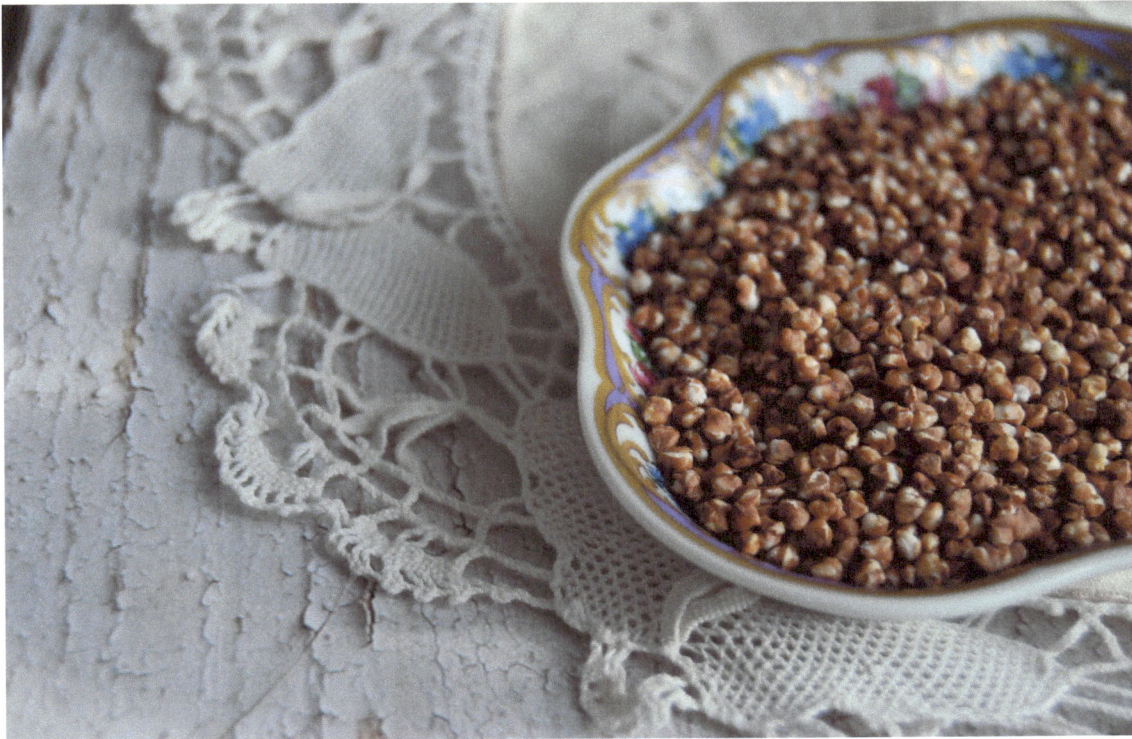

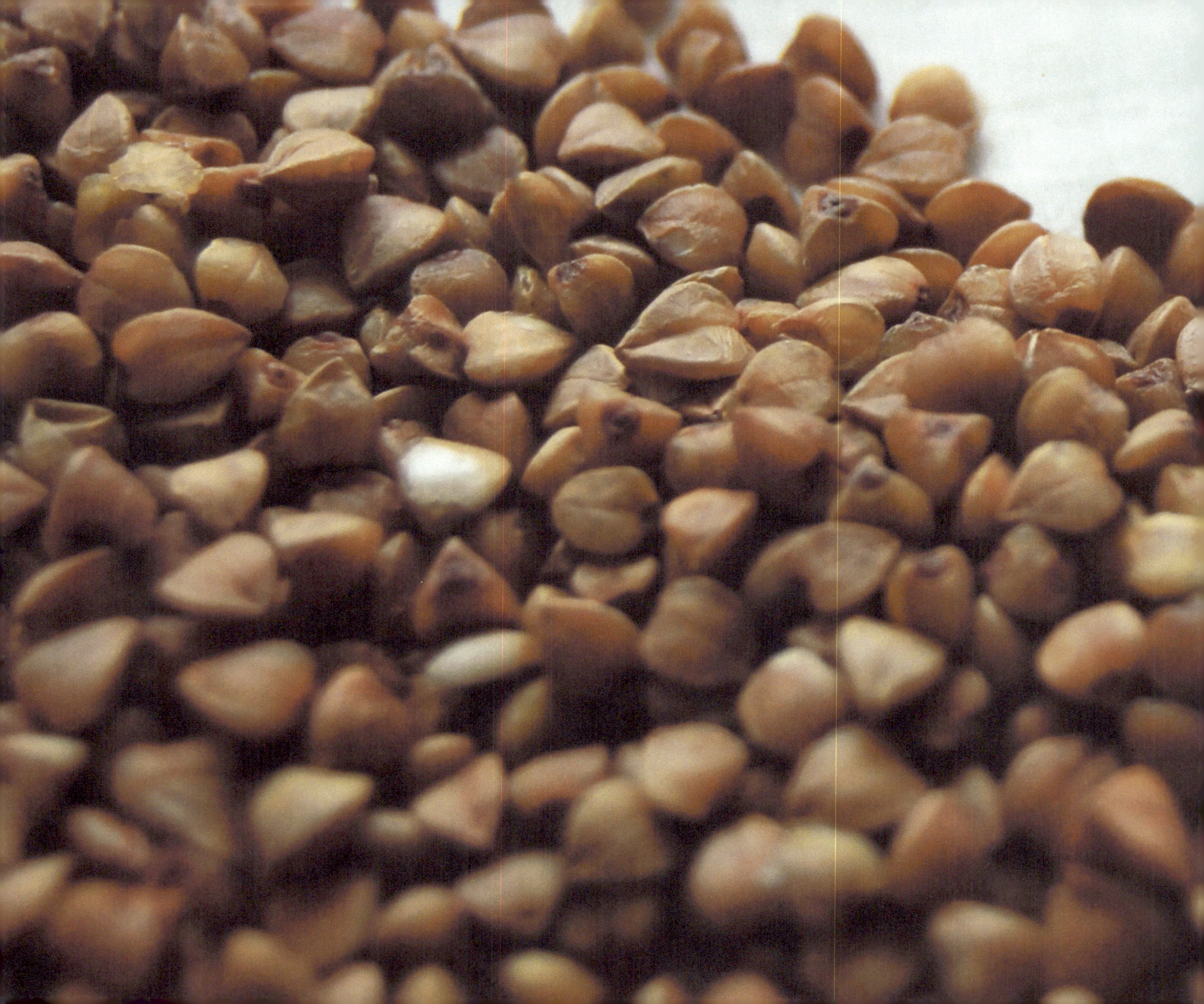

APPETIZERS

Light and airy or hearty and rich, these appetizers are great all year round. Buckwheat appetizers can be served as a part of a big meal or a quick and flavourful snack, and they are sure to add a bold note of comfort and flavour to your dinner routine.

BUCKWHEAT AND MANGO SALAD

Serve this salad with a few slices of fresh baguette at your next summer barbecue.

½ cup (125ml) buckwheat, raw
1 large ripe mango, peeled, diced
¼ cup (60ml) red onion, julienned
½ cup (125ml) red bell pepper, diced
½ cup (125ml) yellow bell pepper, diced
½ cup (125ml) fresh cilantro, chopped

Dressing:
¼ cup (60ml) vegetable oil
3 tbsp lemon or lime juice
1 tsp salt
1 tsp black pepper, ground

Makes 4 servings

Preparation time: 20 minutes

In a medium saucepan cover buckwheat with 1 cup of water and simmer on medium heat until all water is absorbed and buckwheat is tender. Remove saucepan from heat and cool the buckwheat to room temperature. In a large bowl combine buckwheat, mango, red onion, red bell pepper, yellow bell pepper, cilantro. In a small bowl whisk together vegetable oil, lemon juice, salt and pepper. Season the salad with the dressing and serve chilled.

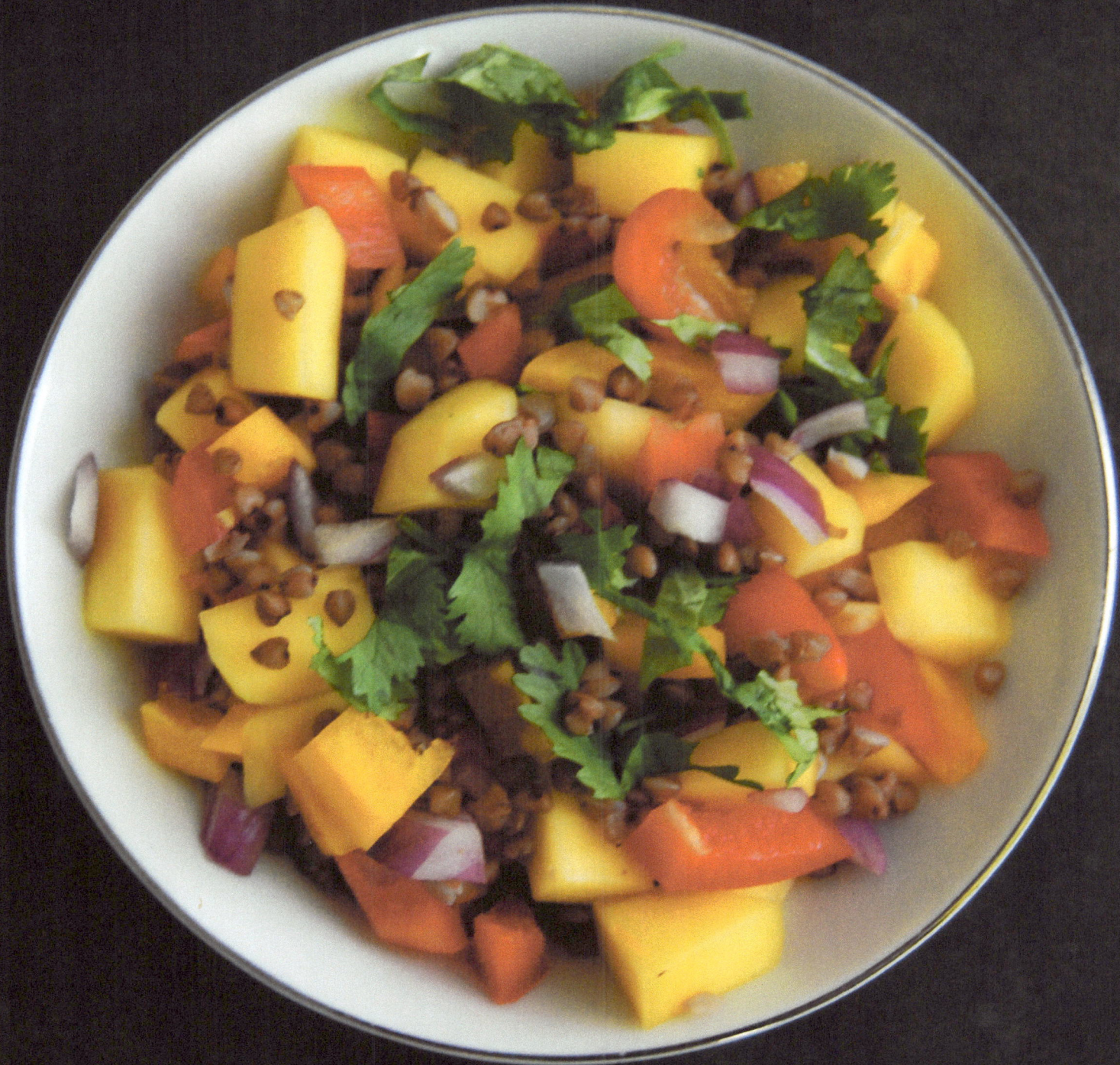

BUCKWHEAT AND VEGETABLE SOUP

After a brisk walk in the park on a frosty weekend you will surely appreciate
a bowl of this soup as a simple and comforting lunch.

2L water
1 medium potato, peeled, diced
1 cup (250ml) leeks, thinly sliced
1 bay leaf
2 black pepper kernels
1-2 tsp (5-10ml) salt
1 tbsp (15ml) butter or vegetable oil
½ cup (125ml) celery root, shredded
½ cup (125ml) celery stalks, thinly sliced
1 large carrot, peeled, shredded
1 small shallot, thinly sliced
½ cup buckwheat uncooked

Bring about 2L of water to a boil in a medium pot. Once the water boils, add the potato and leeks and simmer on low heat for about 10 minutes. Add bay leaf, black pepper and salt to the pot. In a medium skillet or frying pan melt butter and stir-fry celery root, celery stalks, carrot and shallot for about 10 minutes. Add buckwheat to the pot as well as the contents of the frying pan and continue simmering the soup for another 15-20 minutes. Once all vegetables and buckwheat are tender, turn off the heat and serve the soup hot.

Makes 4 servings

Preparation time: 30 minutes

BUCKWHEAT MINT AND PINE NUT SALAD

Serve this salad when you have company over. Goes well with all sorts of flat breads, crackers and a light conversation.

1 cup (250ml) buckwheat
2 cups (500ml) fresh mint leaves
1 cup (250ml) parsley leaves
¼ cup (60ml) pine nuts
2 tbsp (30ml) lemon juice
2 tbsp (30ml) extra virgin olive oil

In a medium saucepan cover buckwheat with 2 cups of water and simmer on medium heat until all water is absorbed and buckwheat is tender. Remove saucepan from heat and cool the buckwheat at room temperature. Rinse the mint and parsley leaves in cold water, pat dry with paper towel and finely chop. In a large salad bowl combine buckwheat, mint, parsley and pine nuts. Season with lemon juice and olive oil and gently mix the salad until all ingredients are well blended.

Makes 4 servings

Preparation time: 30 minutes

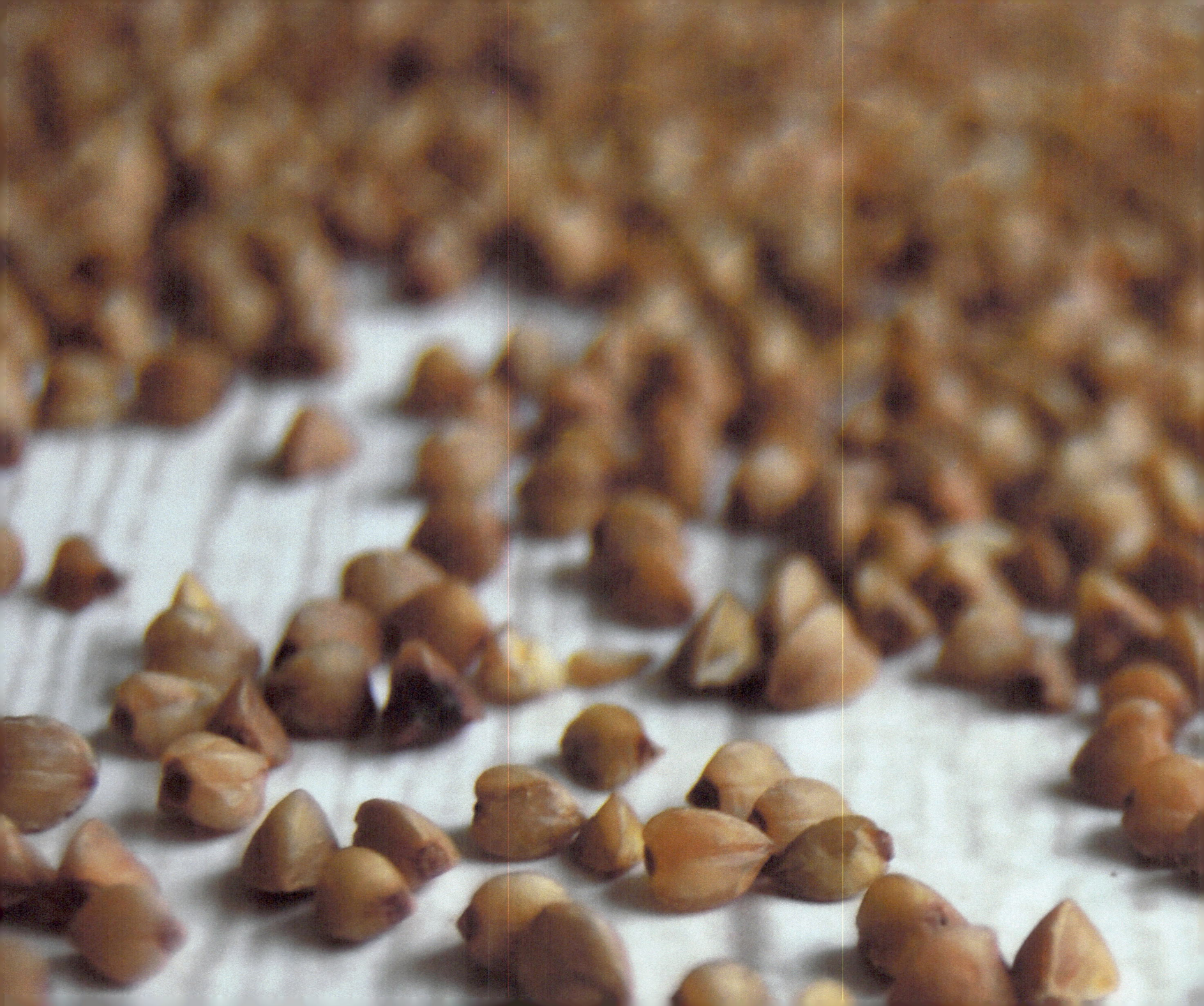

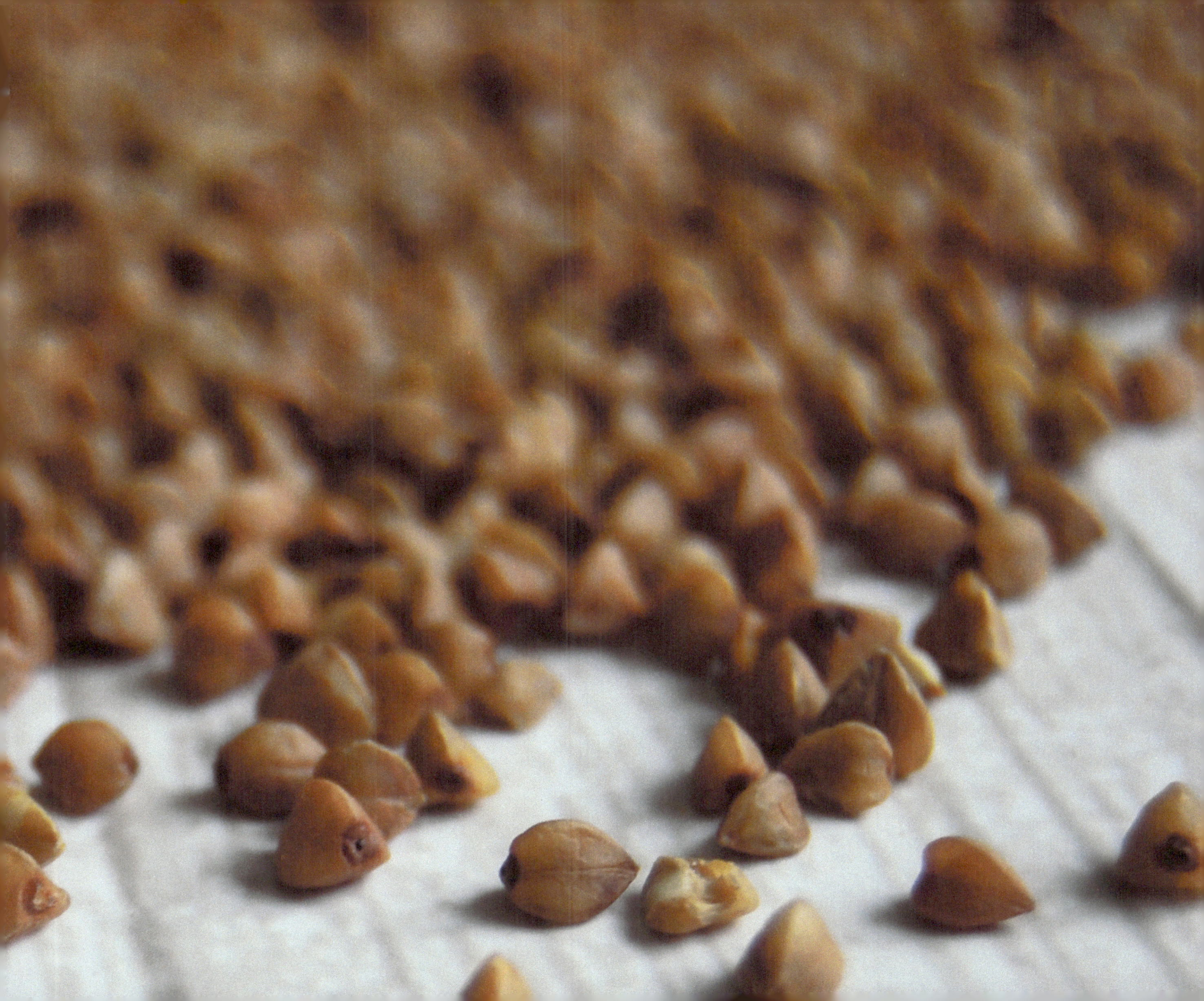

SOBA NOODLE AND VEGETABLE SOUP

Don't be intimidated by the number of ingredients. Broth can be prepared in advance. Delicate noodles and toppings of your choice make this dish especially appealing.

1 large carrot, chopped
1 large parsnip, chopped
1 onion, peeled, whole
3 black pepper kernels whole
1 large bay leaf
1 tsp (5ml) salt
400g buckwheat soba noodles (about 4 bundles)
1 tbsp (15ml) sesame oil or extra virgin olive oil
2/3 cup (225ml) fresh shiitake, enoki and oyster mushrooms, chopped
1 tsp (5ml) canola oil
4 heads baby bock choy, blanched
½ cup (125ml) carrot, shredded
½ cup (125ml) red cabbage, raw, shredded
1 tbsp (15ml) fresh ginger root, peeled, grated
4 green onions, trimmed, finely sliced on the diagonal
2 tsp (10ml) lime juice
2 tbsp (30ml) miso paste
½ tsp (2.5ml) salt
1 cup (250ml) fresh coriander, chopped
2 tbsp (30ml) sesame seeds

In a large pot combine your future broth ingredients - chopped carrot, onion, parsnip, black pepper, bay leaf and salt and cover them all with cold water. The water level should cover the vegetables by about 5-10 cm (2 to 4") while still leaving room at the top of the pot so it doesn't boil over. Cover and bring to a boil. Reduce the heat and simmer for 30-40 minutes skimming off any foam that rises to the top. Once all vegetables are very tender, turn off the heat and let the broth sit for about an hour.

In a separate pot bring to a boil about 2L of water. Drop the soba noodles in boiling water and cook for about 4 minutes until they are soft. Drain the cooked soba noodles and rinse under cold running water to stop them cooking any further. Set aside to drain, then drizzle over a little sesame oil and mix through to prevent the noodles from sticking to each other. Divide the noodles between the four soup bowls.

In a small frying pan panfry the mushrooms with canola oil until golden. Place the mushrooms, bok choy, carrot and red cabbage in equal portions on top of each noodle bowl.

Remove cooked vegetables form the broth. Heat the broth liquid on medium heat and stir in grated ginger, green onions, lime juice, miso paste and salt. Pour the hot broth over the vegetables. Top each bowl with fresh cilantro and sesame seeds and serve.

Makes 4 servings

Preparation time: 1 hour

BUCKWHEAT AND ROASTED VEGETABLE SALAD

Entertaining a big crowd has never been easier. This salad is full of colour and goodness.

1 bunch rainbow carrots
2 red bell peppers chopped
1 red onion sliced in wedges
2 tbsp (30ml) olive oil
¼ cup (60ml) orange juice
1 tsp (5ml) cumin
2 tsp (10ml) fresh ginger, grated
1 garlic clove
1 ½ tbsp (20ml) buckwheat honey
1 cup (250ml) buckwheat uncooked
1 ½ tbsp (20ml) lemon juice
1 cup (250ml) fresh cilantro
1 cup (250ml) parsley fresh
1 cup (250ml) arugula

Preheat oven to 190°C (380°F). Line baking tray with parchment paper. Spread carrots, bell peppers, onion and drizzle with half of oil. Roast the veggies for 15 min. To prepare the glaze for the vegetables whisk together orange juice, cumin, ginger, garlic and honey. Drizzle over half cooked vegetable and continue roasting, turning half way for another 25-30 min. until all vegetables are tender.

In a small saucepan cook buckwheat as described in Simple buckwheat recipe on p.- 31 using 2 cups of water for 1 cup of buckwheat. To prepare the dressing in a small bowl whisk together lemon juice and remaining oil and honey. In a large mixing bowl toss together roasted vegetables (cooled to room temperature), buckwheat, fresh cilantro and parsley. Drizzle with dressing and serve.

Makes approximately 6 portions

Preparation time: 1 hour

BUCKWHEAT AND ROASTED BEET SALAD WITH BALSAMIC AND OLIVE OIL DRESSING AND ARUGULA

Beauty in simplicity is the essence of this salad. A few slices of fresh crusty bread and a drink of your choice and you got yourself a light lunch or brunch all set.

1 cup (250ml) buckwheat, raw
4 large beets
1 cup (250ml) fresh baby arugula
¼ cup (60ml) walnut halves
Dressing:
4 tbsp (60ml) extra virgin olive oil
2 tbsp (30ml) balsamic vinegar
1 tsp (5ml) salt
1 tsp (5ml) ground black pepper

In a medium saucepan cover buckwheat with 2 cups of water and simmer on medium heat until all water is absorbed and buckwheat is tender. Remove saucepan from heat and cool the buckwheat to room temperature.

Place unpeeled beets on a baking tray and bake for about 1 hour at 190°C (370°F), until they can be easily pierced with a knife. Cool them down to room temperature and remove the skins.

To prepare the dressing combine olive oil, balsamic vinegar, salt and black pepper.

Slice beets into thin rounds and arrange on a platter. Top with baby arugula mixed with cooked buckwheat and walnuts. Drizzle with dressing and serve warm or cold.

Makes 4 servings

Preparation time: 1 hour 15 minutes

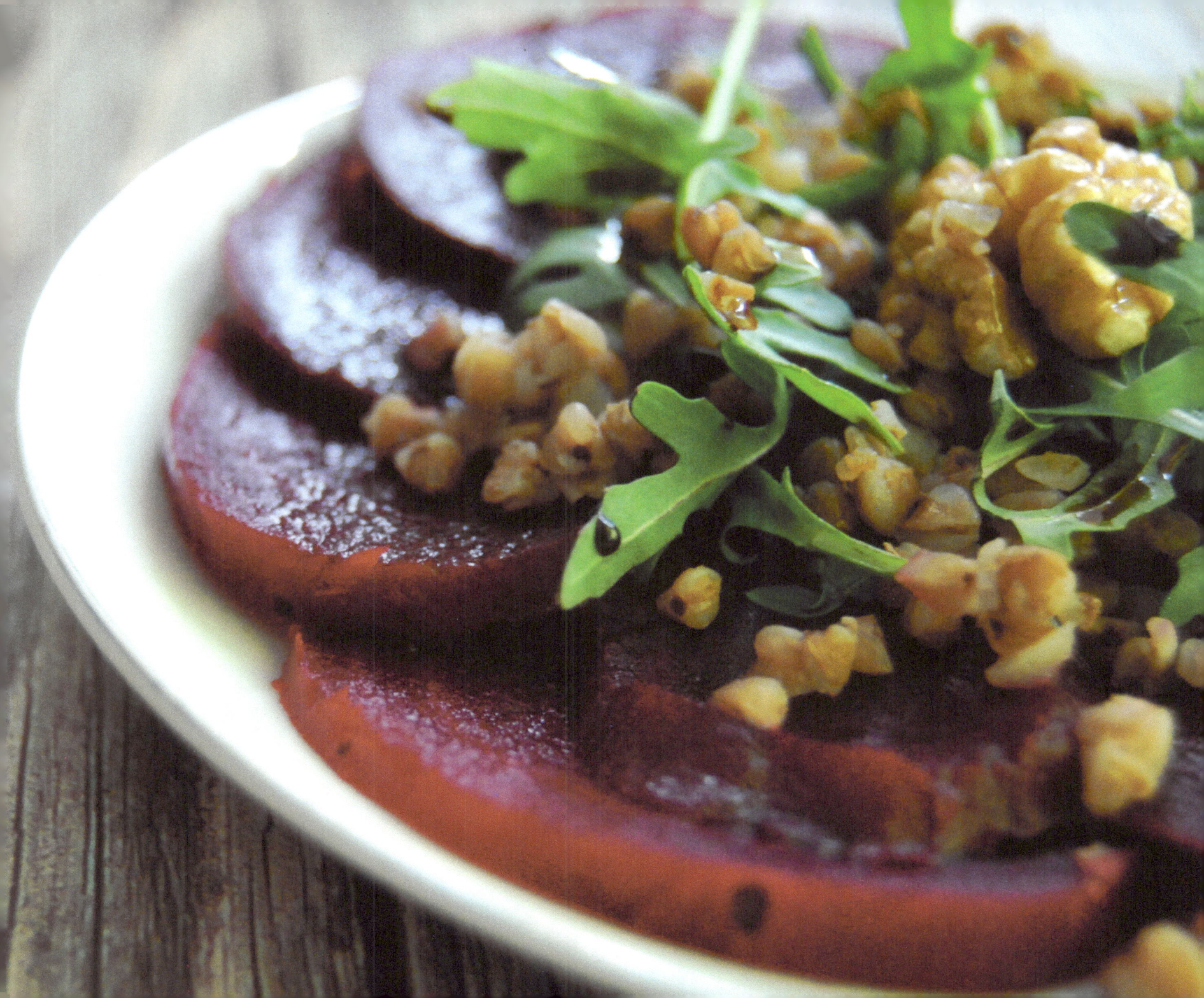

BUCKWHEAT BLINI WITH SMOKED SALMON, SOUR CREAM, SALMON CAVIAR AND DILL

A Russian classic. Serve with literary conversation and some classical music on the side.

½ cup (125ml) all purpose wheat flour
½ cup (125ml) buckwheat flour
4 tsp (60ml) sugar
1 ¼ tsp (7ml) active dry yeast
2 eggs
¼ tsp (2ml) salt
2 cups (500ml) whole milk
3 tbsp (45ml) butter, cut into cubes
2 large eggs, lightly beaten
6 slices of smoked salmon
½ cup (125ml) sour cream
½ cup (125ml) salmon caviar
¼ cup (60ml) fresh dill

Buckwheat in Eastern Europe

Buckwheat is one of the most popular grains in Russia and Ukraine, Russia being the world leader in buckwheat crops. Typically served as boiled grains (similar to rice) as a side dish accompaniment to the main course. Buckwheat flour dishes such as buckwheat blini (see recipe on p.17) are also an integral part of Russian traditional cuisine. In Ukraine pampushki (see recipe on p.21) and korzhik (see recipe on p.25) are also made from buckwheat flour and constitute an important part of the traditional cuisine.

Makes approximately 6 large blinis

Preparation time: 1 hour 30 minutes

In a mixing bowl combine wheat flour with buckwheat flour, sugar, yeast and salt. In a small cup combine milk, butter and heat until butter is melted. Pour warm milk and butter into the flour mix and mix until smooth. Stir in eggs and make sure they are completely incorporated in the dough. Cover the bowl with plastic wrap and let stand in warm corner for about 1 hour until dough doubles in volume.

Stir the dough to deflate, add some more warm milk if it thickens too much. Then poor some dough on the frying pan or crepe maker, spread all over the surface and bake from both sides like regular crepes. Transfer cooked blini onto a ceramic plate and keep in in the oven set on lowest heat to keep warm until you are done baking all of them.

To serve, place some smoked salmon on each blini, fold in quarter and top with sour cream and some salmon caviar. Add some fresh dill on top.

These blinis also could be served as a build-your-own creation where all toppings are set on the table in separate dishes and guests can build their own dish.

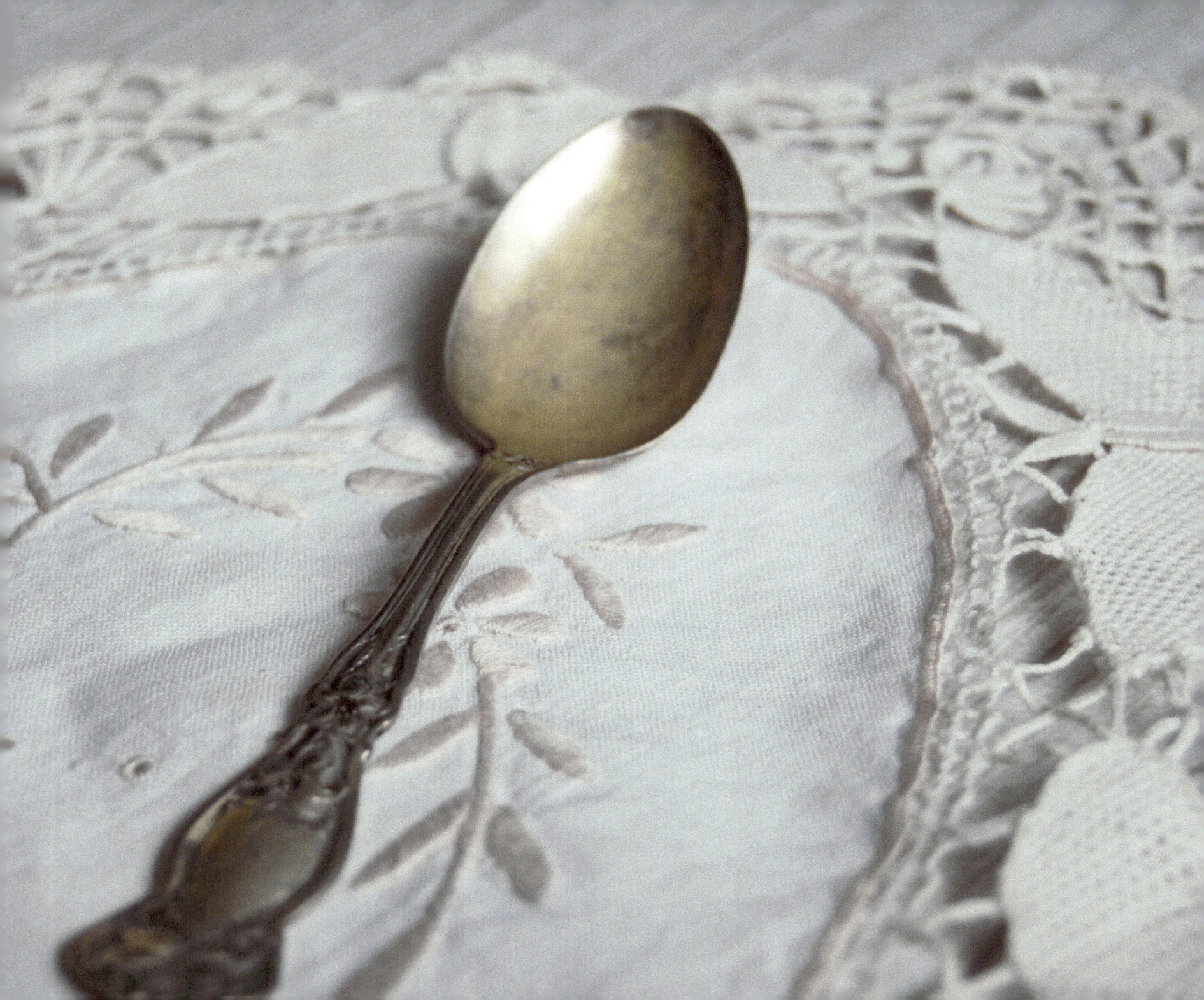

BUCKWHEAT AND MUSHROOM SOUP

This is the soup I usually make in the winter. Rich and hearty, it has a lovely earthy aroma that fills the entire house and makes most welcoming dinner.

1 cup (250ml) brown mushrooms
½ cup (125ml) good quality dried porcini mushrooms
½ cup (125ml) buckwheat
½ cup (125ml) 35% cream
1 tsp (5ml) black pepper
½ tsp (2.5ml) salt
½ cup (125ml) fresh parsley chopped

In a medium bowl cover porcini mushrooms with about 1L boiling water and let stand for about 30 minutes Peel the brown mushrooms, brushing them with a cloth or paper towel from dry debris. Slice them and place in a large saucepan. Add porcini mushrooms and liquid where they soaked and cook on medium low heat for about 20 minutes Then add the buckwheat, salt and pepper and continue cooking for another 20 minutes until buckwheat and porcini mushrooms are all tender. Add the cream and transfer soup into a blender or food processor. Puree the soup in a blender and transfer it into a serving dish or pot. If soup turns out too runny for your liking you can add about 1 tbsp of corn starch mixed in ¼ cup cold water and heat the soup, stirring occasionally until it thickens.

To serve top each bowl with freshly chopped parsley.

Makes 4 servings

Preparation time: 50 minutes

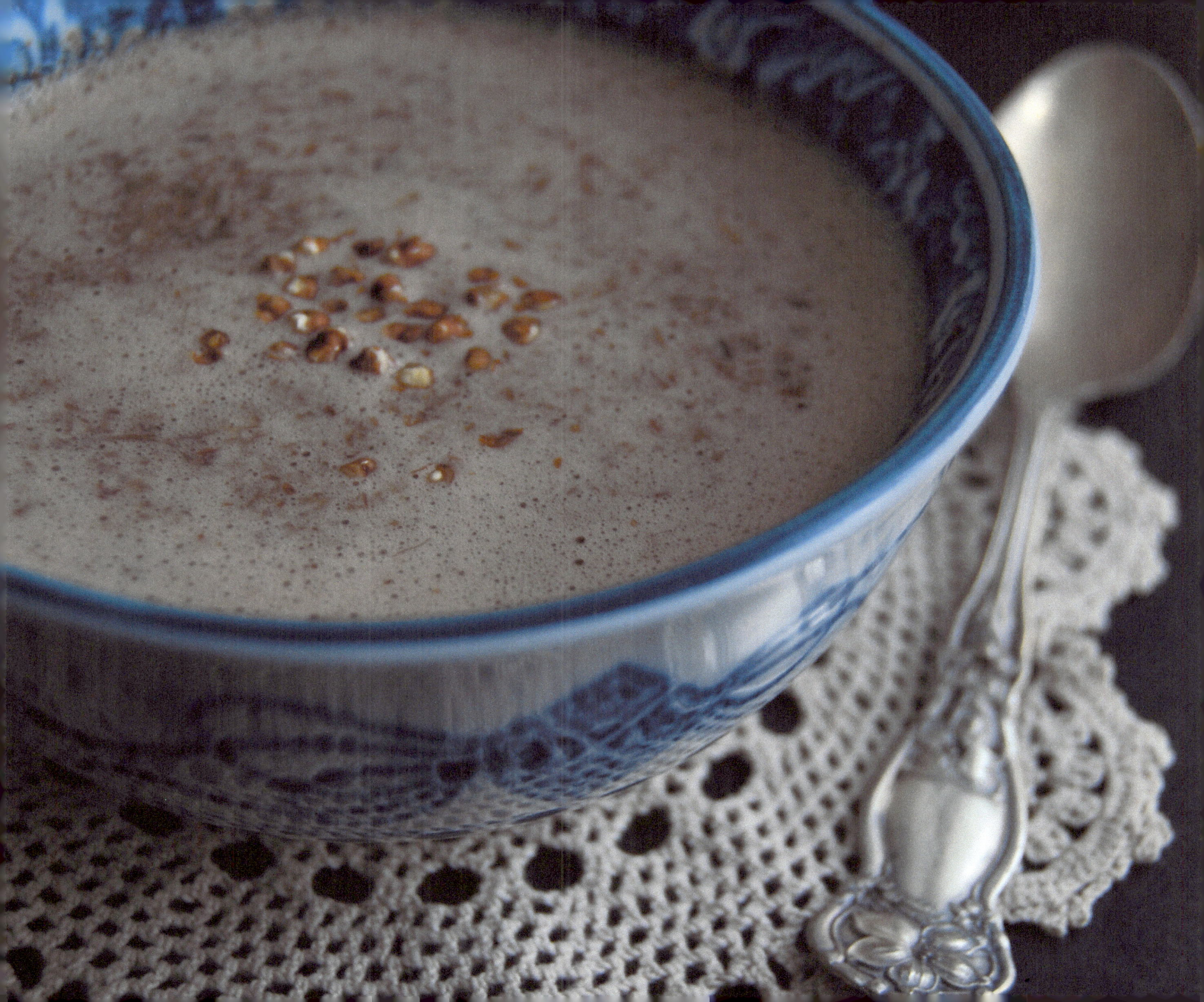

PAMPUSHKI WITH GARLIC DIPPING SAUCE

Pampushki is a traditional Ukrainian dish. It can be made with wheat or buckwheat flour and is typically served as a light appetizer before main course.

2 ⅔ cups (725ml) buckwheat flour
3 tsp (15ml) quick rise yeast
1 tsp (5ml) salt
1 tbsp (15ml) sunflower oil
⅔ cup (150ml) water
Sauce:
3 cloves garlic
¼ cup (60ml) unrefined sunflower oil
1 tsp (5ml) salt
1 tsp (5ml) ground coriander

In a mixing bowl combine warm water yeast, a quarter of the total amount of flour, blend it all well and let rise for about 30 min. in a warm spot on the counter. Add remaining flour, sugar, salt, sunflower oil and knead into soft dough. Cover it with clean tea towel and let rise for another hour. Preheat the oven to 360°F (180°C). Once dough rises again, carefully knead it again, roll the dough into small balls approximately the size of a walnut. Set the balls onto a baking sheet lined with parchment paper. Let them sit at room temperature for about 25-30 minutes and increase in size. Bake at 360°F (180°C) for about 10 minutes until wooden pick comes out clean.

To prepare the dipping sauce in a ceramic small bowl rub together minced garlic with salt, add sunflower oil and rub again until smooth, Stir in ground coriander and serve in a small dish as a dipping sauce for pampushki.

Makes approximately 20 pampushki

Preparation time: 2 hours

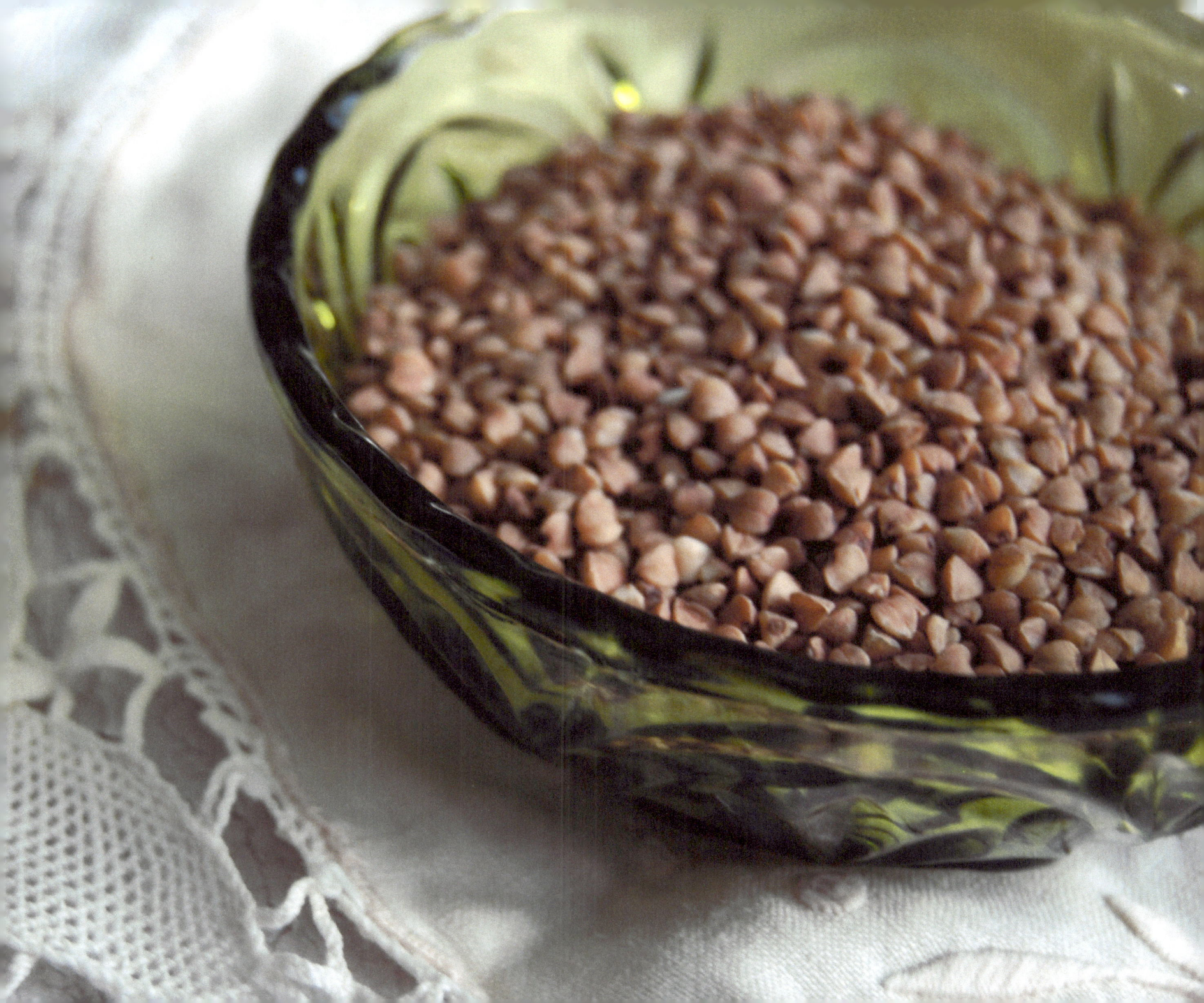

PORTOBELLO MUSHROOM CAPS STUFFED WITH BUCKWHEAT, PARSLEY AND GRUYERE CHEESE

Great idea for a festive get together or a summer barbeque appetizer.

4 large Portobello mushrooms
1 tbsp (15ml) olive oil
½ cup (125ml) buckwheat
2 cloves garlic
⅓ cup (75ml) fresh parsley, chopped
⅓ cup (75ml) Gruyere cheese shredded

Carefully remove stems from the mushrooms. Brush away any debris from caps surface with a paper towel and place them upside down on a baking sheet, lined with parchment paper.

Preheat the oven to 200°C (400°F).

Cook the buckwheat as described in the Simple buckwheat recipe using 2 cups water per 1 cup buckwheat. In a small frying pan heat 1 tbsp of oil with minced garlic for 1-2 minutes Stir in cooked buckwheat, take off heat and stir in parsley and gruyere cheese.

Top the mushroom caps with buckwheat mixture and bake at 200°C (400°F) for about 15-18 minutes until cheese is melted and a bit roasted on top. Serve hot.

Makes 4 servings

Preparation time: 1 hour

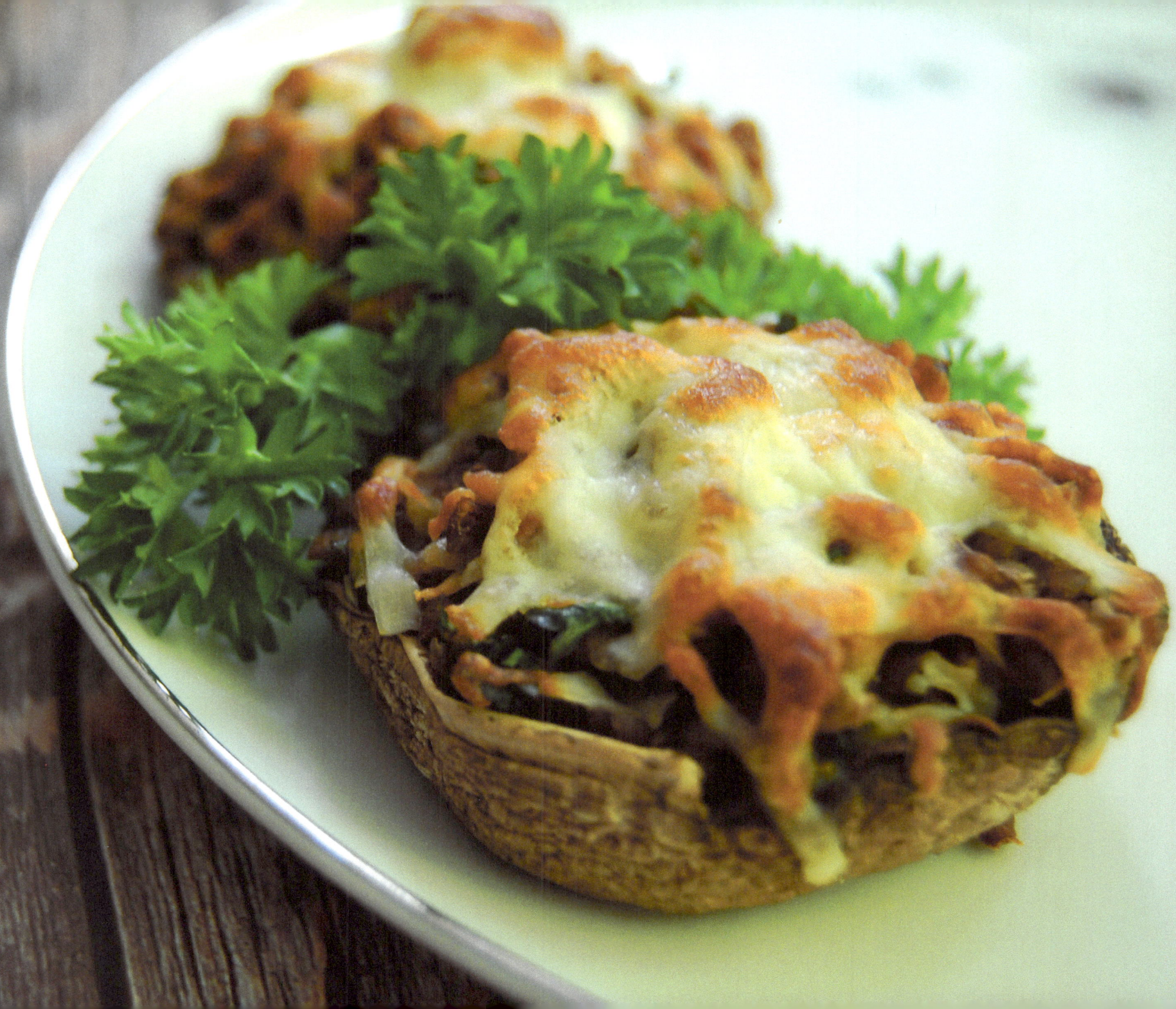

BUCKWHEAT KORZHIK WITH DOUBLE SMOKED BACON

Korzhik is a Ukrainian version of a pastry similar to scone, easy to make and fantastic in flavour.
Serve them as a side to your favourite soup and see smiles light up everywhere.

⅔ cup (225ml) double smoked bacon cut into small cubes
1 ¼ cup (310ml) buckwheat flour
¾ cup (180ml) all purpose wheat flour
1 ½ tsp (7.5ml) baking powder
1 tsp (5ml) salt
1 tsp (5ml) freshly ground black pepper
¼ cup + 1 tbsp (75ml) cold unsalted butter cubed
2-3 tbsp (60-45ml) ice cold water

Why do we combine buckwheat flour with wheat flour?

As buckwheat flour is naturally gluten free in some recipes just buckwheat flour alone will not produce necessary elasticity of the dough or batter. So wheat flour is added to help achieve desired texture of the dough. If you wish to have a completely wheat free recipe, consider adding equivalent of 1 or 2 eggs of a powdered egg replacer instead of wheat flour.

Makes 16 portions

Preparation time: 1 hour

In a frying pan, toss the bacon and heat on medium heat until pieces become semi transparent. Remove bacon from the pan and set aside.

In a large mixing bowl, combine together wheat and buckwheat flour, baking powder, black pepper and salt. Cut in the cold butter with hand or fork in order to form pea sized lumps of flour covered cold butter. Carefully drizzle over some ice cold water while mixing the dough, until dough forms a uniform lump and no loose flour remains. Knead in the bacon bits. Wrap the dough into plastic wrap and refrigerate for about 30 minutes. Preheat the oven to 200°C (400°F). After refrigeration roll out the dough into a round about ½ inch thick. Using a cookie cutter or glass rim cut out the round scones and pace them on a baking sheet lined with parchment paper. Bake the korzhik for about 15- 25 minutes. Remove immediately from the sheet and serve hot or at room temperature.

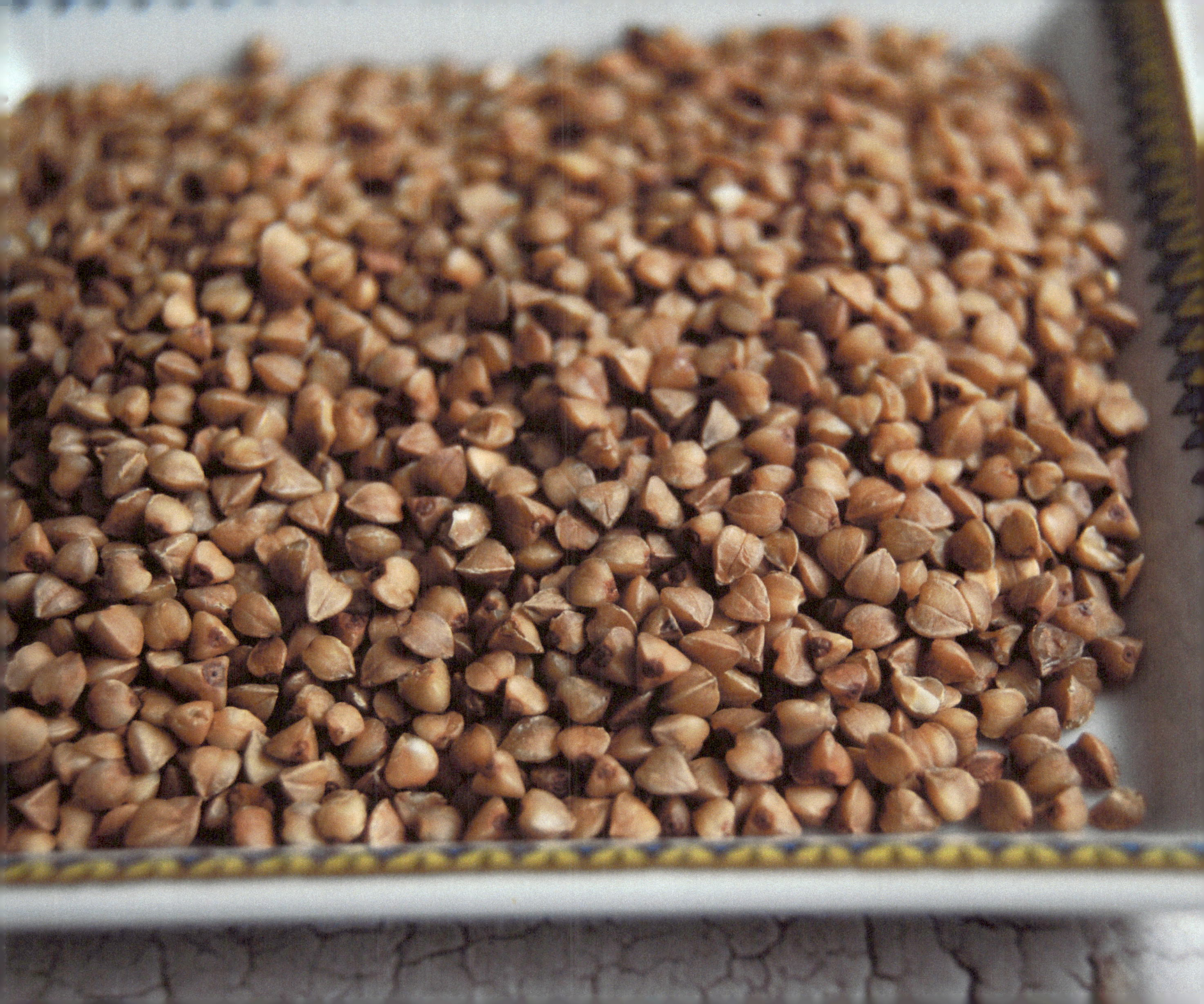

BUCKWHEAT TABBOULEH

Perfect for hot summer days when you can't be bothered to turn on the stove. Cook up the buckwheat in the morning then use it later when you are ready for a light but flavourful meal. The more mint you put in it the better.

2 cups (500ml) buckwheat, uncooked
1L water
1 tsp (5ml) salt
1 bunch of fresh parsley, minced
1 bunch fresh mint, minced
2 large ripe tomatoes, diced
1 large cucumber, diced
1 large shallot, minced
5 tbsp (75ml) extra virgin olive oil
4 tbsp (60ml) lime juice
1 tsp (5ml) salt
1 tsp (5ml) ground black pepper

Place a large dry frying pan on medium heat. Let it warm up then add the buckwheat and heat it up, stirring constantly. After about 4-5 minutes, pleasant aromas will develop and grains will begin to crackle. Continue stirring and heating until grains start popping up like corn. As soon as this process starts, remove pan from heat and transfer buckwheat into a deep saucepan. Cover with full amount of water, add salt and place on medium heat to cook. Can cook with lid on or off, for about 20 minutes. Stirring is not necessary. As soon as all water is absorbed by the grains and they become tender, take the saucepan off the heat and cool off buckwheat.

In a large salad bowl, combine parsley, mint leaves, tomatoes, cucumbers and shallot. Top up with cold cooked buckwheat and stir well. Season with olive oil, lime juice, salt and black pepper and stir again. Serve chilled.

Makes 6 portions

Preparation time: 30 minutes

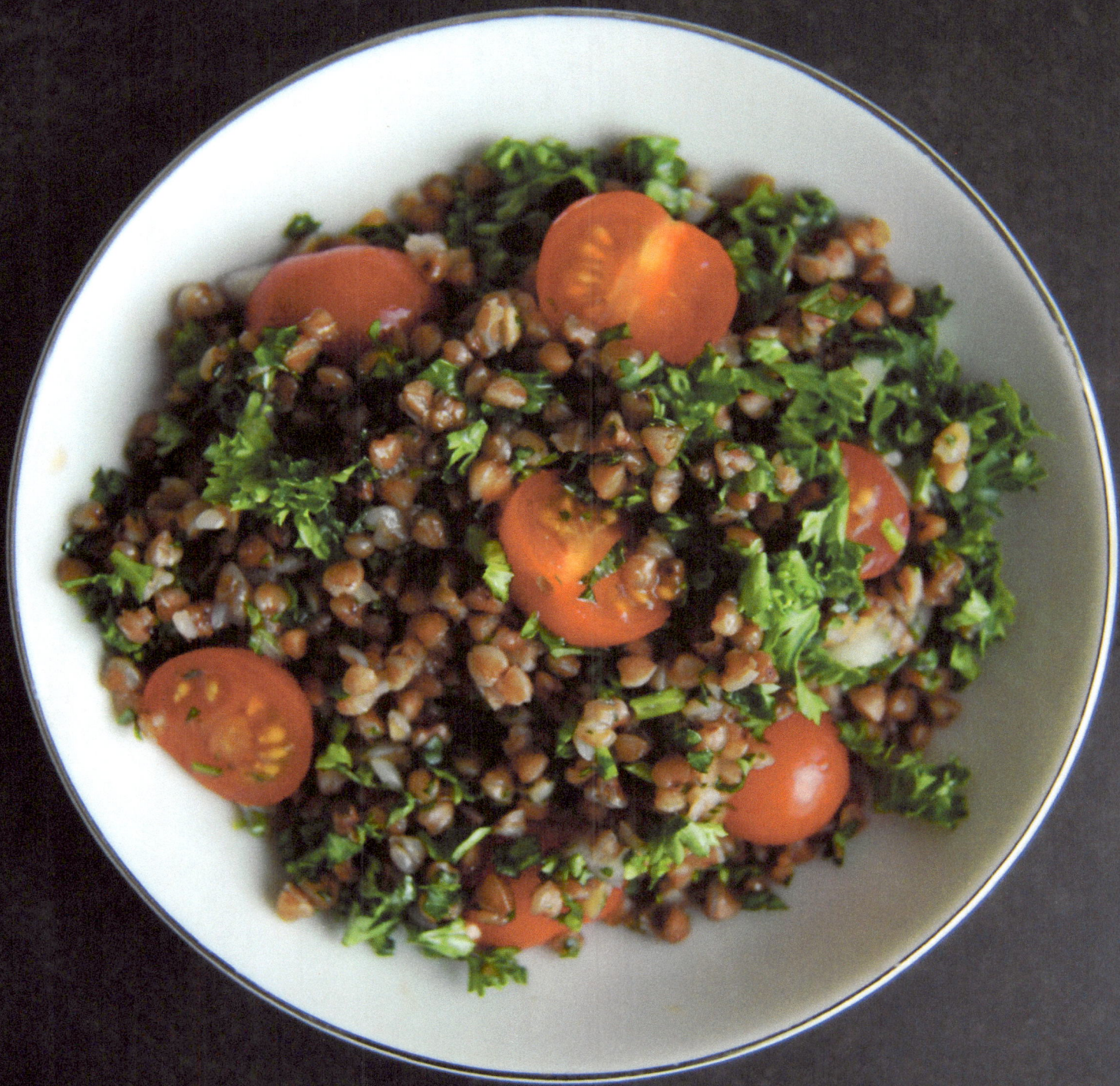

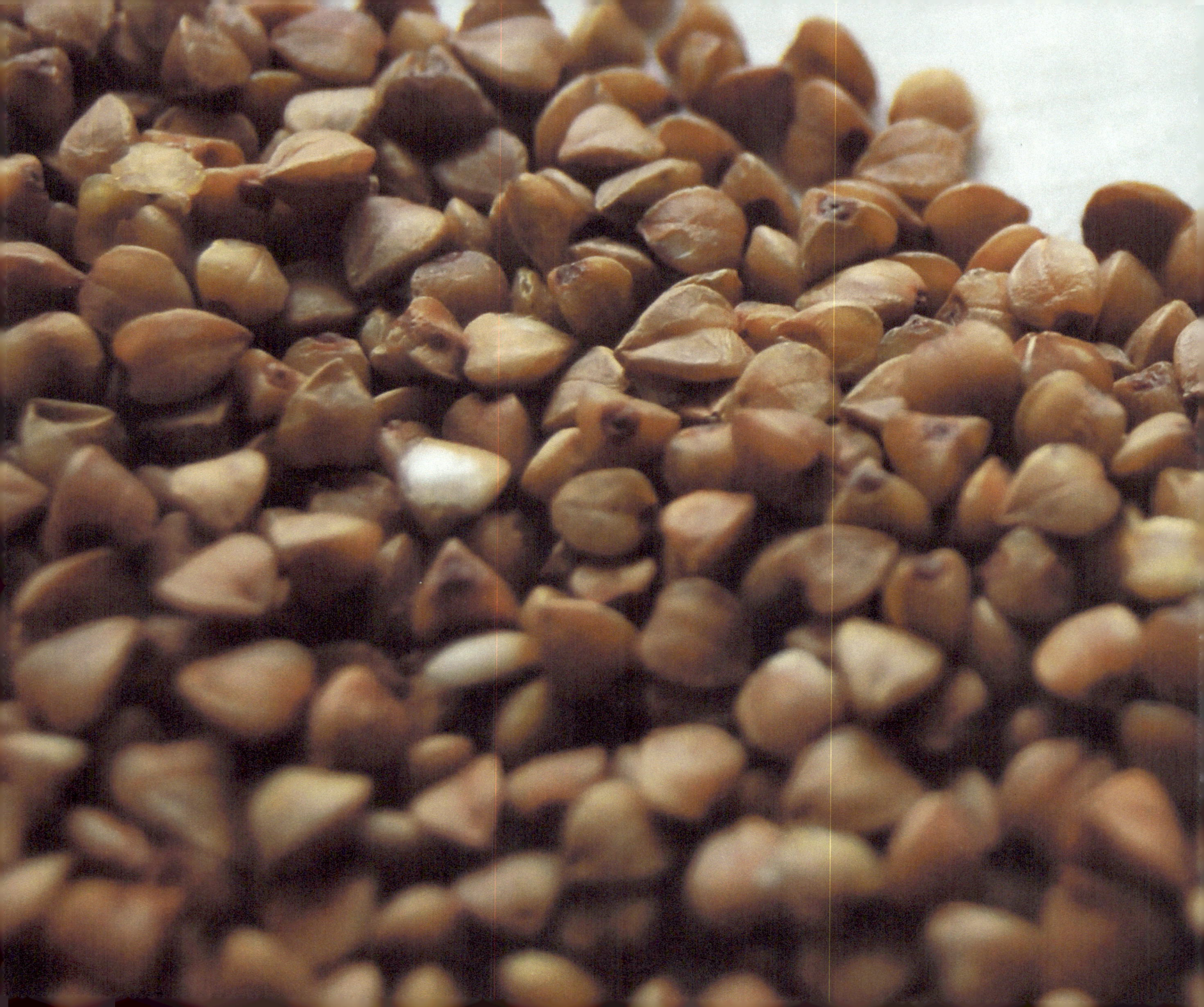

MAIN COURSE

From my heart to yours.

Directly from the oven onto your favourite plate.

Soak in those aromas and flavours.

SIMPLE BUCKWHEAT

This is the base recipe to be used anywhere in this book where cooked buckwheat is required. It makes a simple and delicious side dish to any main course.

2 cups (500ml) buckwheat
4 cups (1L) water
3 tbsp (45ml) butter (optional)
1 tsp (5ml) salt

Place a large dry frying pan on medium heat. Let it warm up then add the buckwheat and heat it up, stirring constantly. In about 4-5 minutes pleasant aroma will develop and grans will begin to crackle. Continue stirring and heating until grains start popping up like corn. As soon as this process starts, remove pan from heat and transfer buckwheat into a deep saucepan. Cover with full amount of water, add salt and place on medium heat to cook. Can cook with lid on or off, for about 20 minutes. Stirring is not necessary. As soon as all water is absorbed by the grains and they become tender, take the saucepan off the heat and stir in butter (if using).

Makes 4 servings

Preparation time: 25 minutes

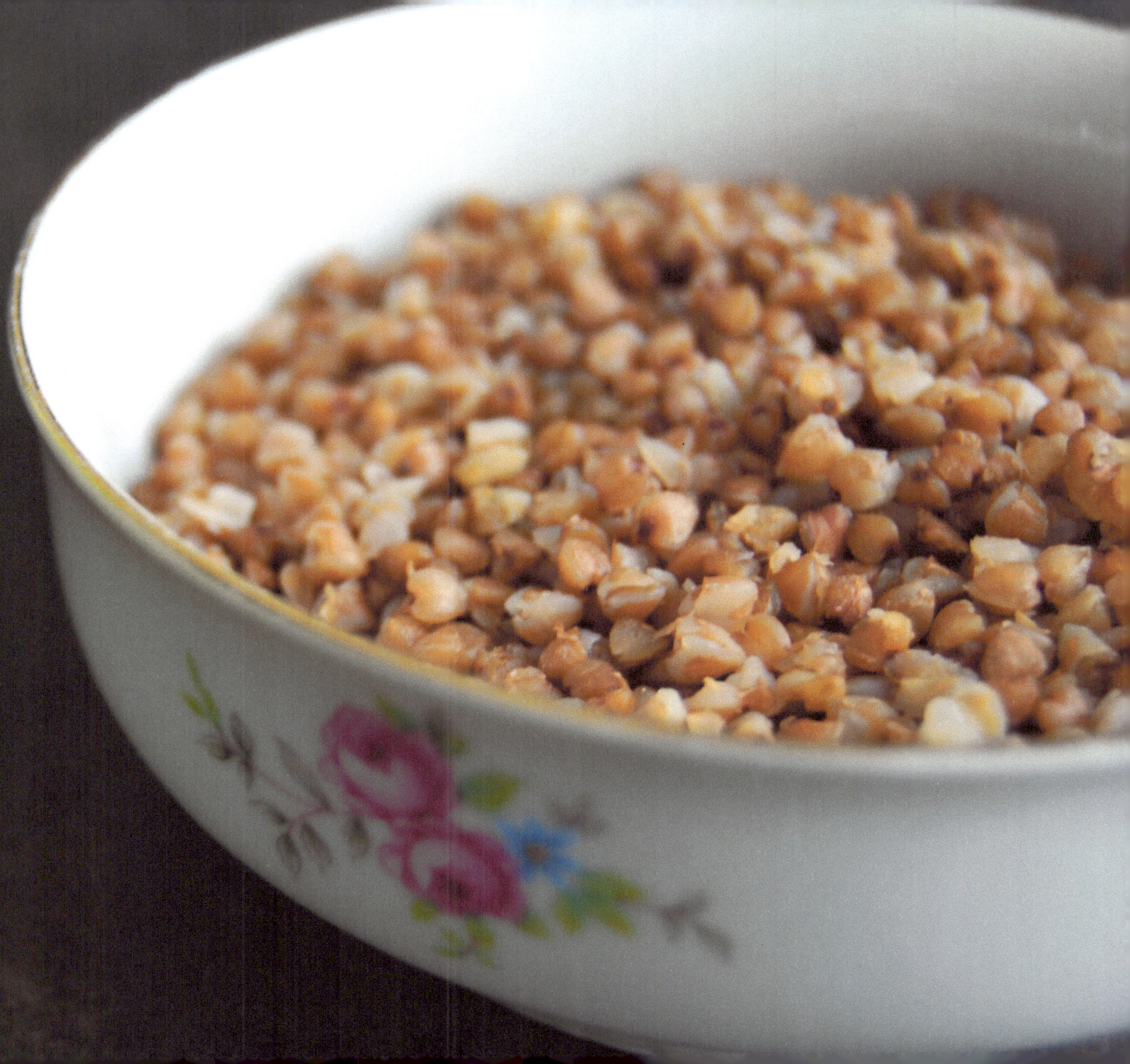

BUCKWHEAT AND MUSHROOM MEDALLIONS

Elegant, flavourful and easy to make these medallions work well on their
own, as a side for fish or meat or in a burger. Give it a try!

1 cup (250ml) buckwheat, raw
1 cup (250ml) oyster mushrooms, minced
1 tsp (5ml) vegetable oil
1 egg
⅓ cup (75ml) flour
1 tsp (5ml) salt
1 tsp (5ml) chili spice mix
2 tsp (10ml) ground black pepper
3 tbsp (45ml) vegetable oil
⅓ cup (75ml) sour cream
¼ cup (60ml) fresh dill

In a medium saucepan, cover buckwheat with 2 cups of water and simmer on medium heat until all water is absorbed and buckwheat is tender. Remove saucepan from heat and cool the buckwheat to room temperature. Pan fry the oyster mushrooms with 1 tsp vegetable oil until golden brown, set aside. In a large bowl, combine buckwheat, mushrooms, egg, flour, salt, chili spice mix and black pepper. Mix everything together to obtain sticky batter. Put a drop of vegetable oil on your hands, take a spoonful of batter and form a round medallion. Heat the vegetable oil in a large skillet or frying pan and pan fry the medallions in small batches from both sides, about 5-10 minutes per batch. Serve hot with a dollop of sour cream and some fresh dill.

Note: Try these medallions as a vegetarian burger.

Makes 4 servings

Preparation time: 45 minutes

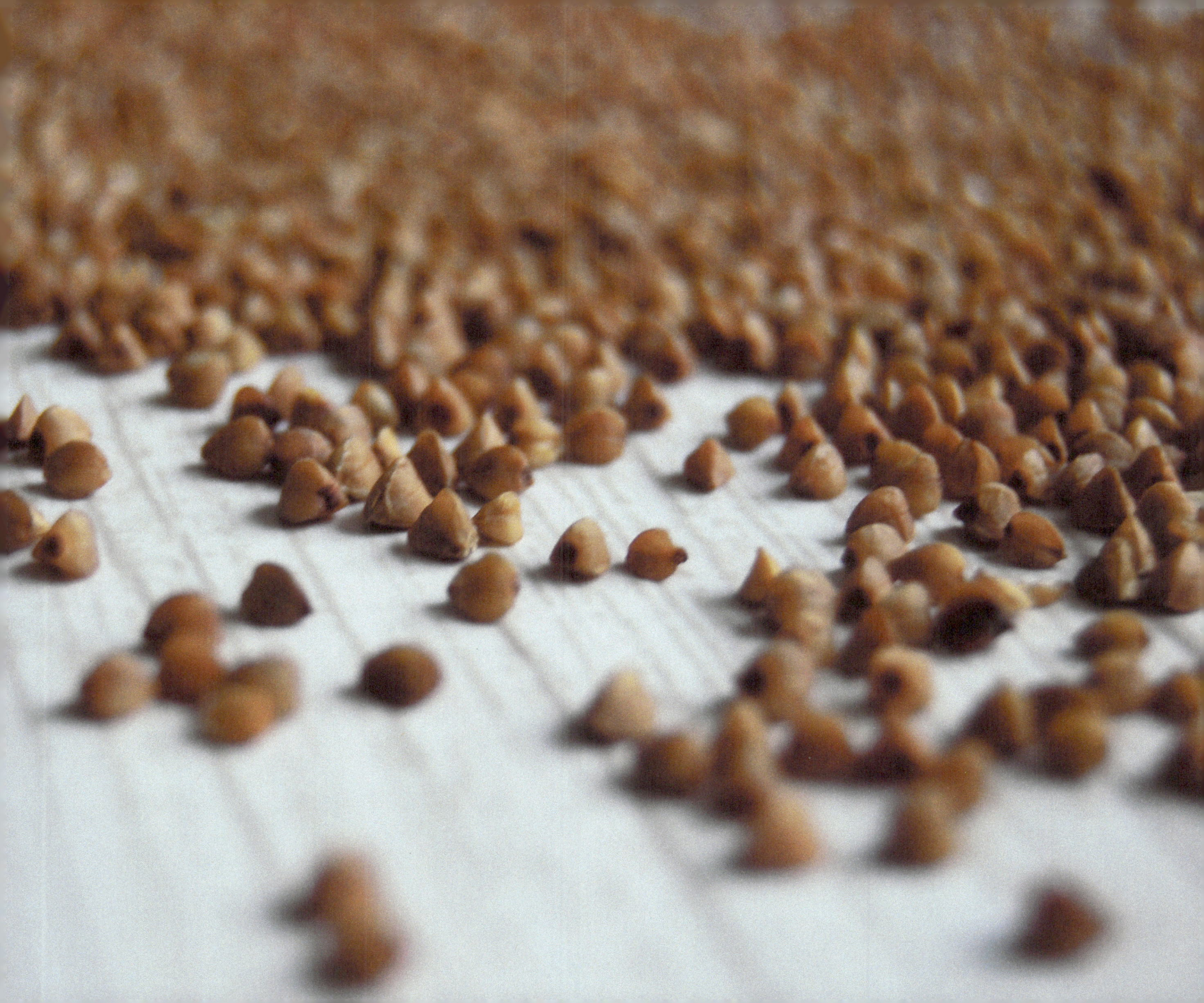

RUSSIAN KASHA - BUCKWHEAT WITH WILD MUSHROOMS AND SHALLOTS

This dish is a Russian traditional dish with a light twist. Traditionally wild foraged mushrooms are used. Store bought are perfectly fine too. Serve on its own or as a fantastic side kick to your favourite meat.

2 tbsp (30ml) extra virgin olive oil
1 cup (250ml) oyster mushrooms, diced
½ cup (125ml) chanterelle mushrooms, diced
2 medium shallots, sliced
2 cups (500ml) buckwheat, raw
1 tsp (5ml) salt
1 tsp (5ml) ground black pepper

In a small skillet, heat the olive oil on medium heat. Add mushrooms and shallots and stir-fry until both mushrooms and shallots become light brown.

In a medium size saucepan, combine 2 cups of buckwheat with 4 cups of cold water and simmer on medium-low heat for about 20-25 minutes until all water is absorbed and buckwheat is tender. Stir in the mushrooms and shallots into the buckwheat, season with salt and pepper and serve hot.

Note: for stronger mushroom flavour, add 2 tbsp of finely crushed dry porcini mushrooms to water in which buckwheat is cooked. You can also add some white truffle oil to give an extra nice kick to the dish.

Makes 4 servings

Preparation time: 35 minutes

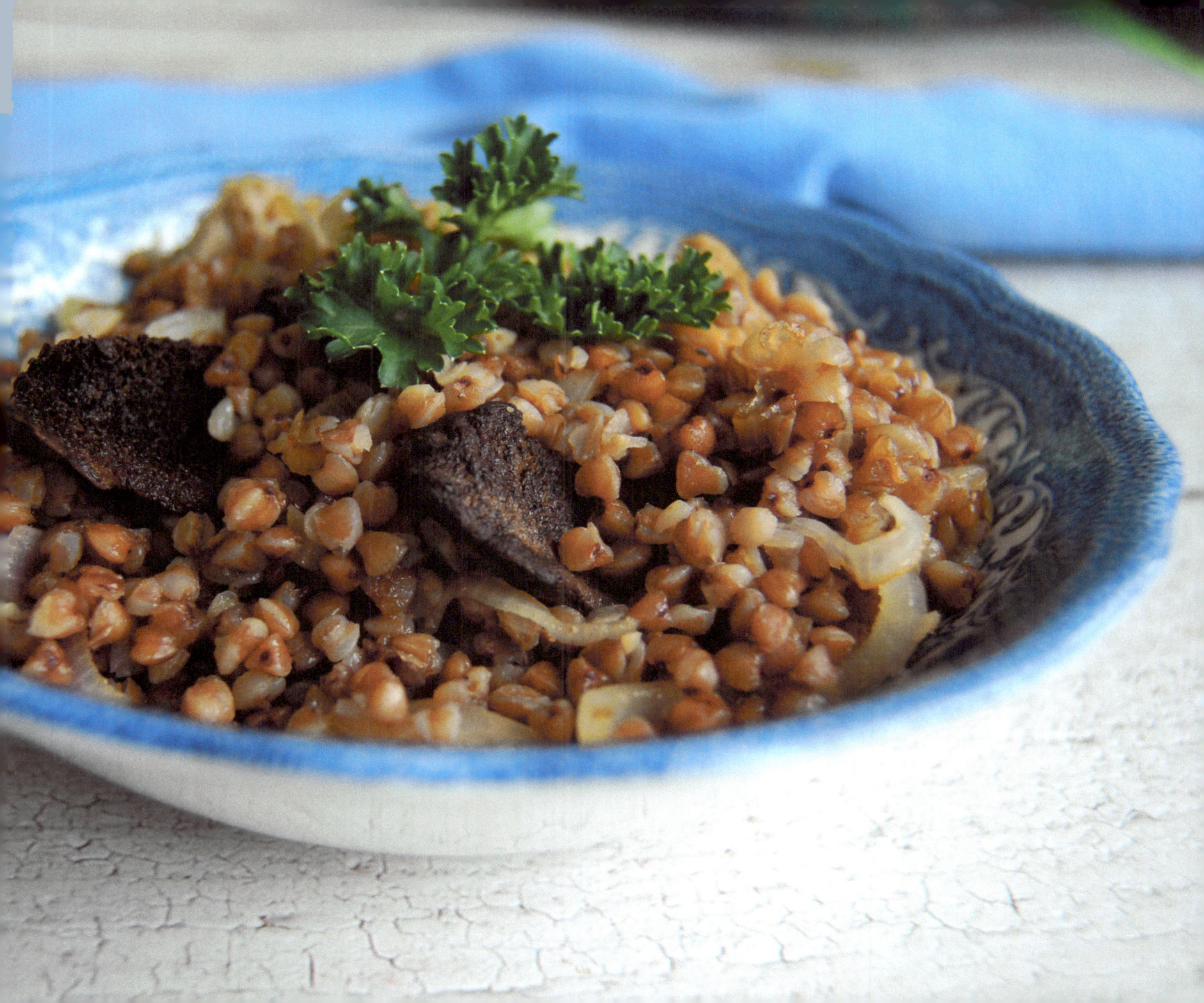

SOBA NOODLE STIR FRY
WITH VEGETABLES, MUSHROOM AND BEEF

Silky noodles, colourful vegetables and a big flavour punch. Oh so fast and delicious!

Sauce:
½ cup (125ml) soy sauce
4 tbsp (60ml) sugar
2 tsp (10ml) garlic
4 tbsp (60ml) sesame seed oil
½ tsp (2.5ml) black pepper

400 g buckwheat soba noodles (about 4 bundles)
1 tbsp (15ml) vegetable oil, divided
3 cups (750ml) beef cut into strips for stir frying
⅓ cups shiitake mushrooms, sliced
1 medium carrot, julienned
1 cup (250ml) red bell pepper, julienned
1 cup (250ml) broccoli, small florets
1 cup (250ml) corn kernels, canned
½ cup (125ml) green onion, cut into thin diagonal
    slices
½ cup (125ml) fresh cilantro

Makes 4 servings

Preparation time: 25 minutes

In a small saucepan on low heat, combine together soy sauce and sugar until sugar is completely dissolved. Add sesame oil, garlic and black pepper, stir ad set aside.

Place buckwheat noodles into a pot with about 2L boiling water and cook for about 4 minutes until tender. Drain the cooked noodles and rinse under cold running water to stop them cooking any further. Add 1 tbsp vegetable oil, stir and set the noodles aside. In a deep skillet or wok heat 1 tbsp vegetable oil and add beef, cook while stirring for about 4 minutes. Add mushrooms, carrot, red pepper, broccoli, corn and continue stir-frying for another 5-8 minutes until mushrooms and beef are cooked through. Add green onion, cilantro, soba noodles and sauce, mix well and take the skillet off the heat. Divide the noodle and vegetable mix into 4 bowls and serve hot.

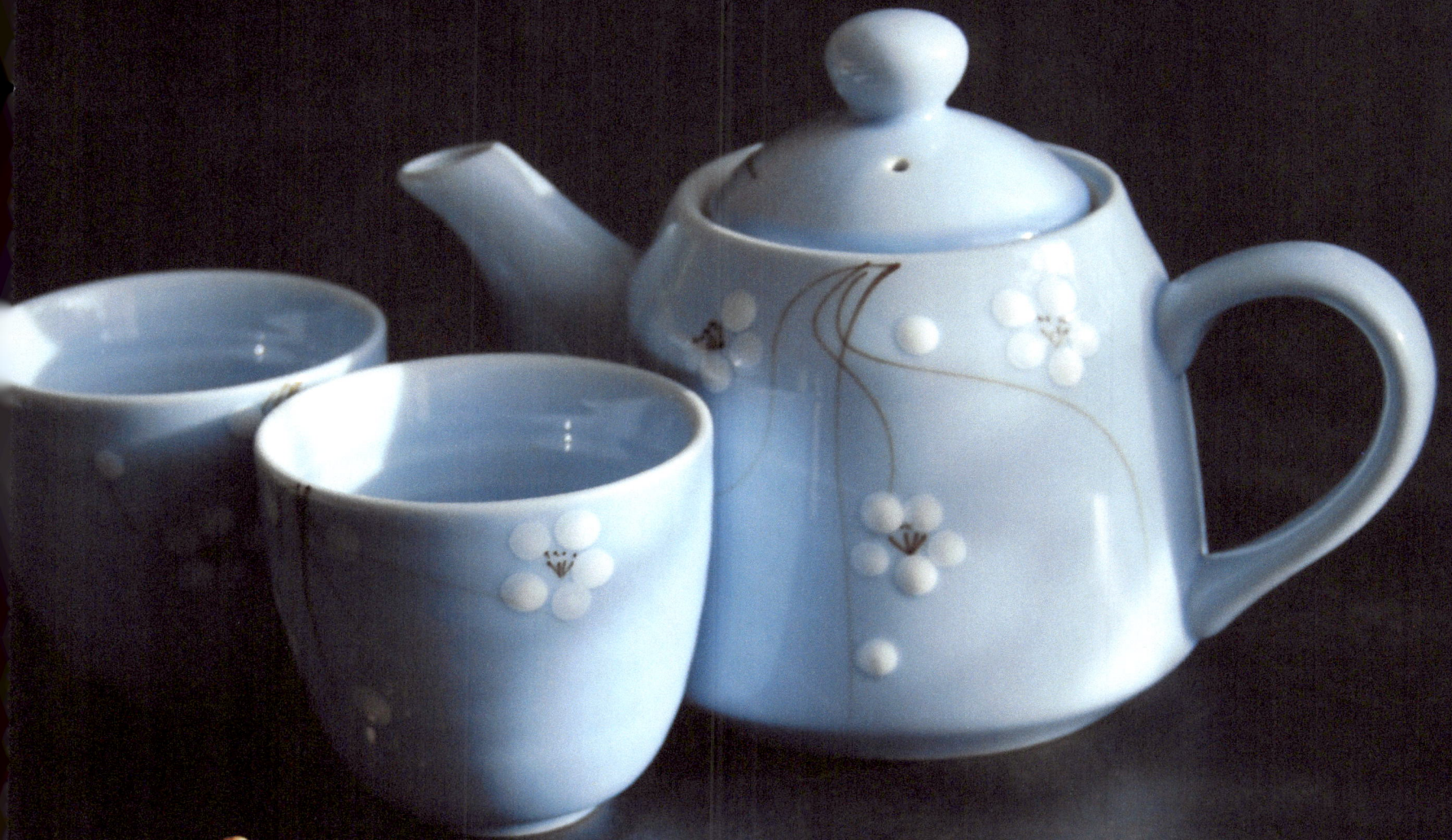

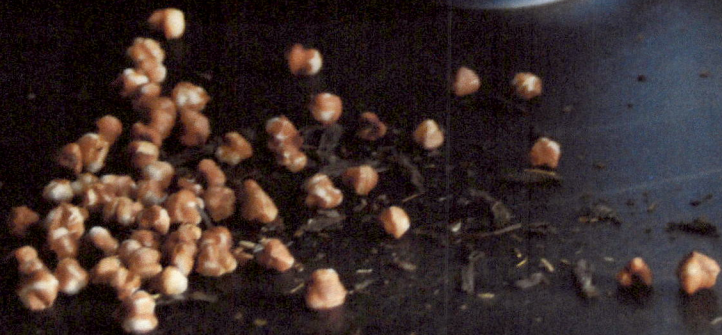

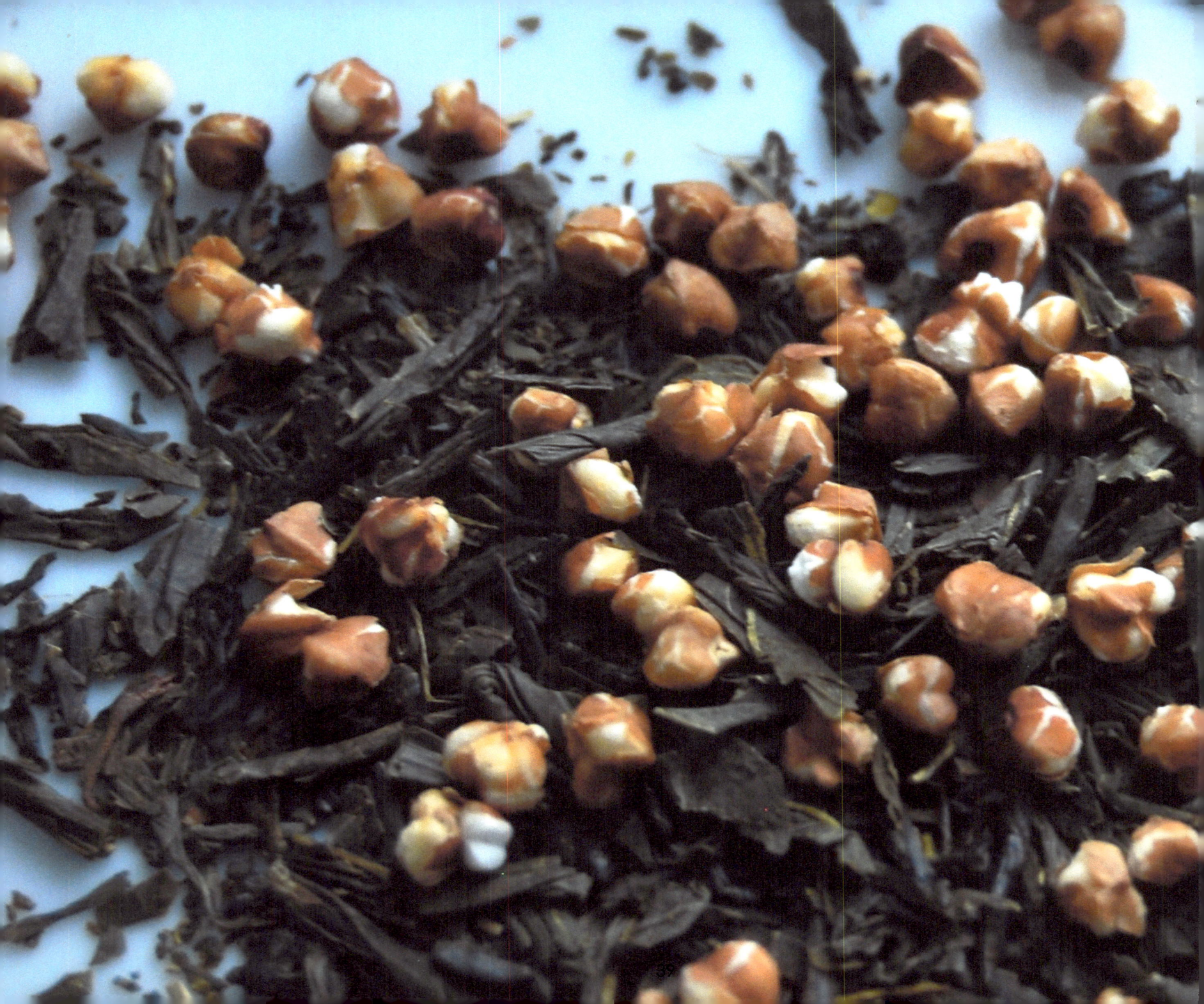

Buckwheat tea

In Japan there is a variety of tea called soba-cha, a tea made with roasted buckwheat kernels with nutty mellow flavour. You can make your own by combining roasted buckwheat kernels from simple buckwheat recipe on p. 31 with some fine Japanese green tea in a proportion of 2 parts roasted buckwheat to 1 part green tea. Brew as you would regular green tea.

BUCKWHEAT ZUCCHINI FRITTERS

Delicious on their own or as a side dish or as a really funky veggie burger
served in a bun with your favourite sauce and toppings.

1 cup (250ml) buckwheat, raw
½ cup (125ml) zucchini, shredded
1 egg
⅓ cup (75ml) flour
1 tsp (5ml) salt
½ tsp (2.5ml) nutmeg
2 tsp (10ml) ground black pepper
3 tbsp (45ml) vegetable oil
⅓ cup (75ml) sour cream

In a medium saucepan, cover buckwheat with 2 cups of water and simmer on medium heat until all water is absorbed and buckwheat is tender. Remove saucepan from heat and cool the buckwheat to room temperature. In a large bowl combine buckwheat, zucchini, egg, flour, salt, nutmeg and black pepper. Mix everything together to obtain sticky batter. Heat the vegetable oil in a large skillet or frying pan and spoon the batter to from several fritters at a time. Cook from both sides, about 5 minutes per batch. Serve hot with a dollop of sour cream.

Makes 4 servings

Preparation time: 45 minutes

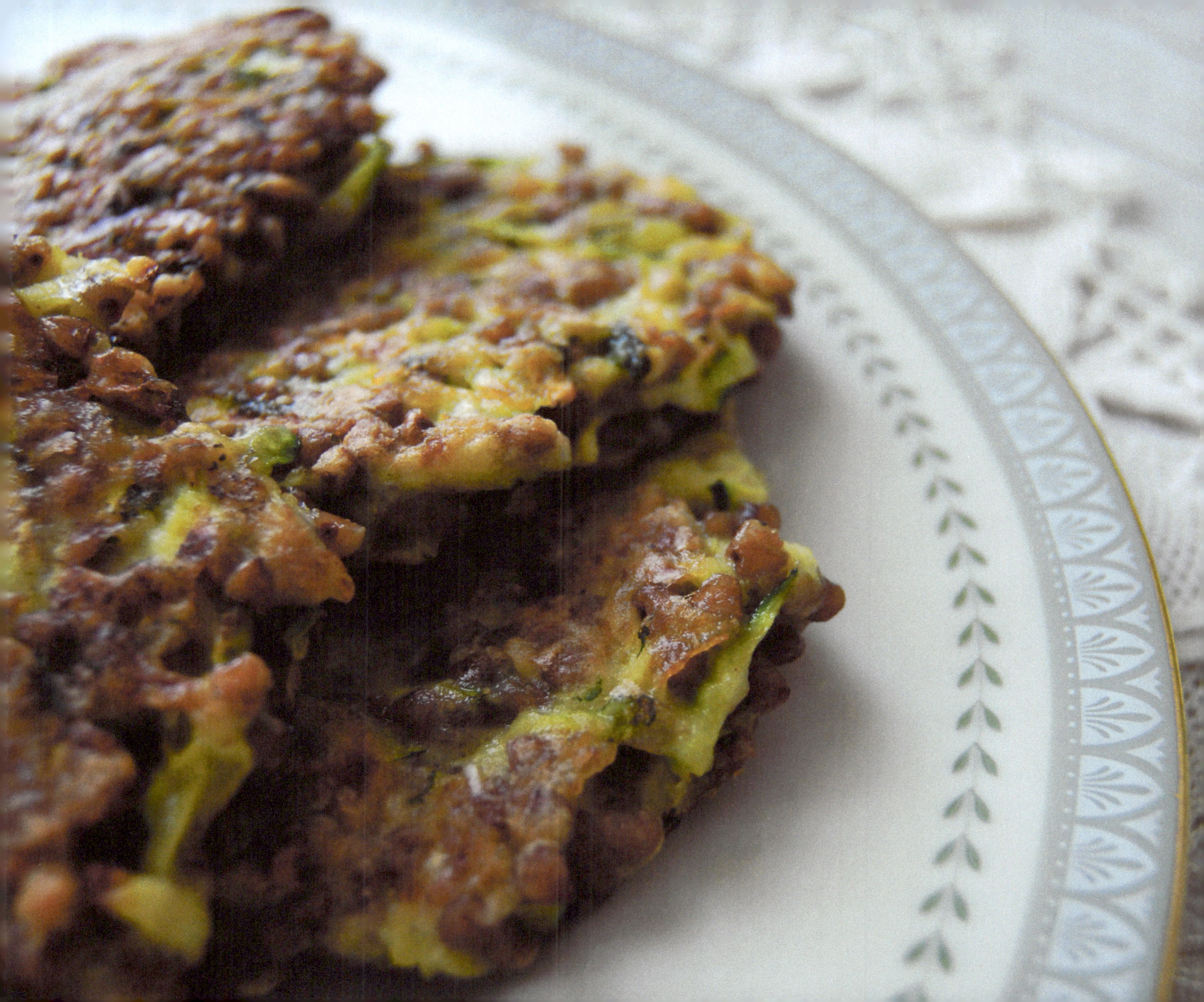

BUCKWHEAT AND BUTTERNUT SQUASH WITH HERBS

Autumn comfort food at its best. Sweet and nutty flavours unite to give the optimal degree of satisfaction.

1 cup (250ml) buckwheat
2 cups (500ml) butternut squash, diced
1 tsp (5ml) herbes de Provence
⅓ cup (75ml) vegetable or chicken broth
¼ cup (60ml) 35% whipping cream
1 tsp (5ml) salt

Preheat the oven to 200°C (400°F).

In a medium saucepan, cover buckwheat with 2 cups of water and simmer on medium heat until all water is absorbed and buckwheat is tender. Remove saucepan from heat and cool the buckwheat to room temperature.

Place butternut squash in a deep oven proof dish. Pour the broth on the bottom of the pan. Season with herbes de Provence, cover with lid and bake at 200°C (400°F) for 30-40 minutes until tender. Place the squash into a bowl, add cream, salt to taste and mash with a potato masher to obtain smooth puree. Carefully fold in the buckwheat. Serve hot.

Makes 4 servings

Preparation time: 1 hour

FRENCH-STYLE
BUCKWHEAT SAVOURY PIE

This is a version of Far Breton de sarrasin – a traditional French dish prepared with buckwheat flour. Far Breton can be sweet or savoury. Rustic looking and loaded with flavour this pie goes very well with a crisp fresh salad and a cup of cider.

½ cup (125ml) buckwheat flour
½ cup (125ml) wheat all purpose flour
½ tsp (2.5ml) baking powder
2 eggs
¼ cup (60ml) salted butter, melted
⅓ cup (75ml) water
1 leek stalk
1 shallot
⅓ cup (75ml) double smoked bacon, diced
⅓ cup (75ml) gruyere cheese
1 tsp (5ml) salt
1 tsp (5ml) fresh ground black pepper

French buckwheat

Wonderful buckwheat also happens to be part of classic French cuisine. The region of Brittany on the Atlantic shore of France is especially rich in buckwheat dishes. They use the flour to prepare galettes (see recipe p.89) – a type of large crepes or pancakes and sweet or savoury pies (see recipe on p.44)

Makes 1 pie

Preparation time: 20 minutes

Preheat the oven to 375°F (200°C).

In a mixing bowl, whisk together eggs, buckwheat flour, baking powder and melted butter. Add water gradually to obtain smooth dough.

In a frying pan, heat up bacon until it becomes crisp, remove them and stir fry leek and shallot in bacon grease for about 2-4 minutes until just a bit tender. Incorporate bacon bits, leeks and onion into the dough. Stir in gruyere cheese and pour the dough into a well greased pie baking dish (preferably ceramic).

Bake for about 30 minutes until toothpick inserted in the middle comes out with no dough sticking to it.

Cool down the pie then slice and serve warm with fresh salad on the side.

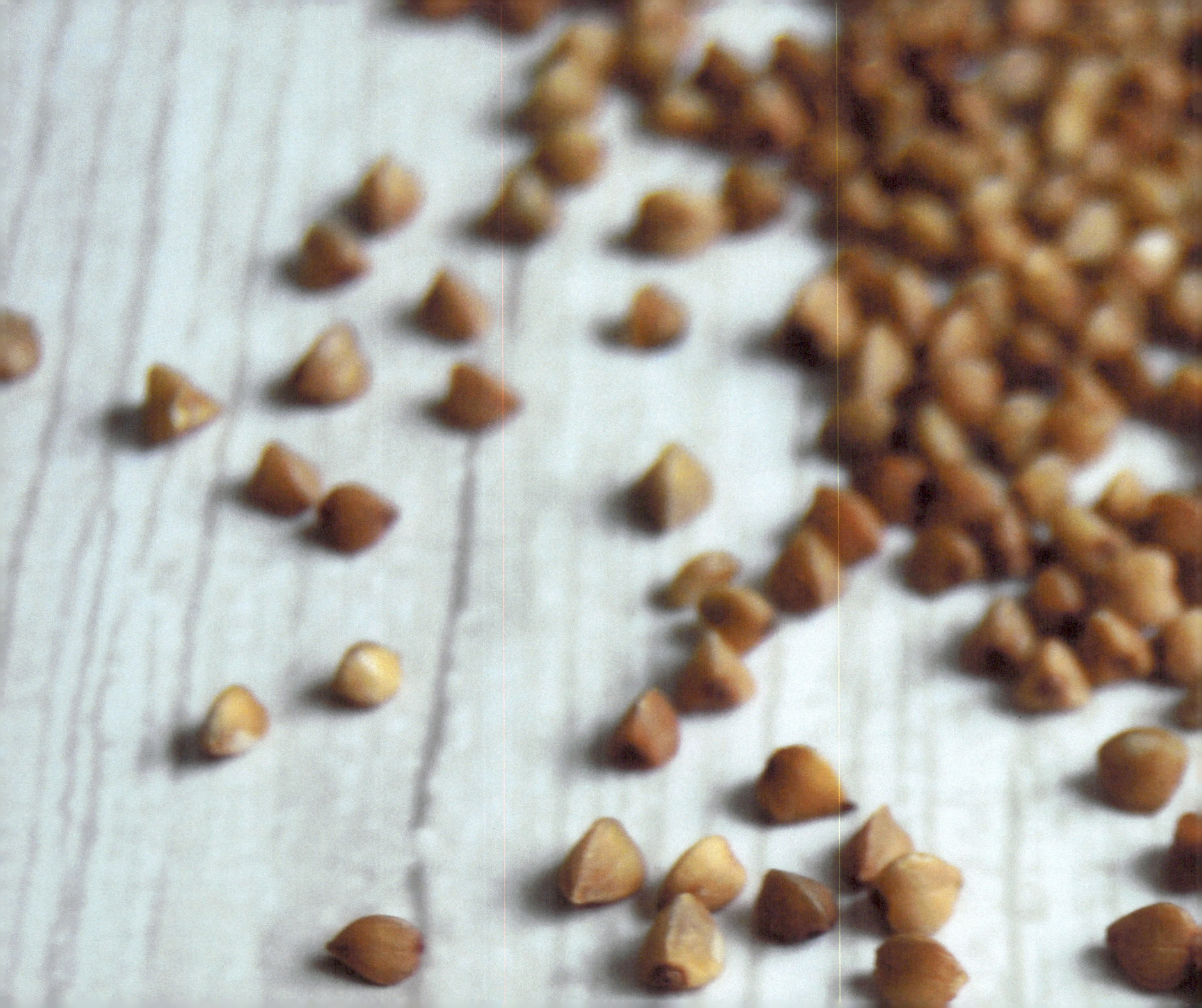

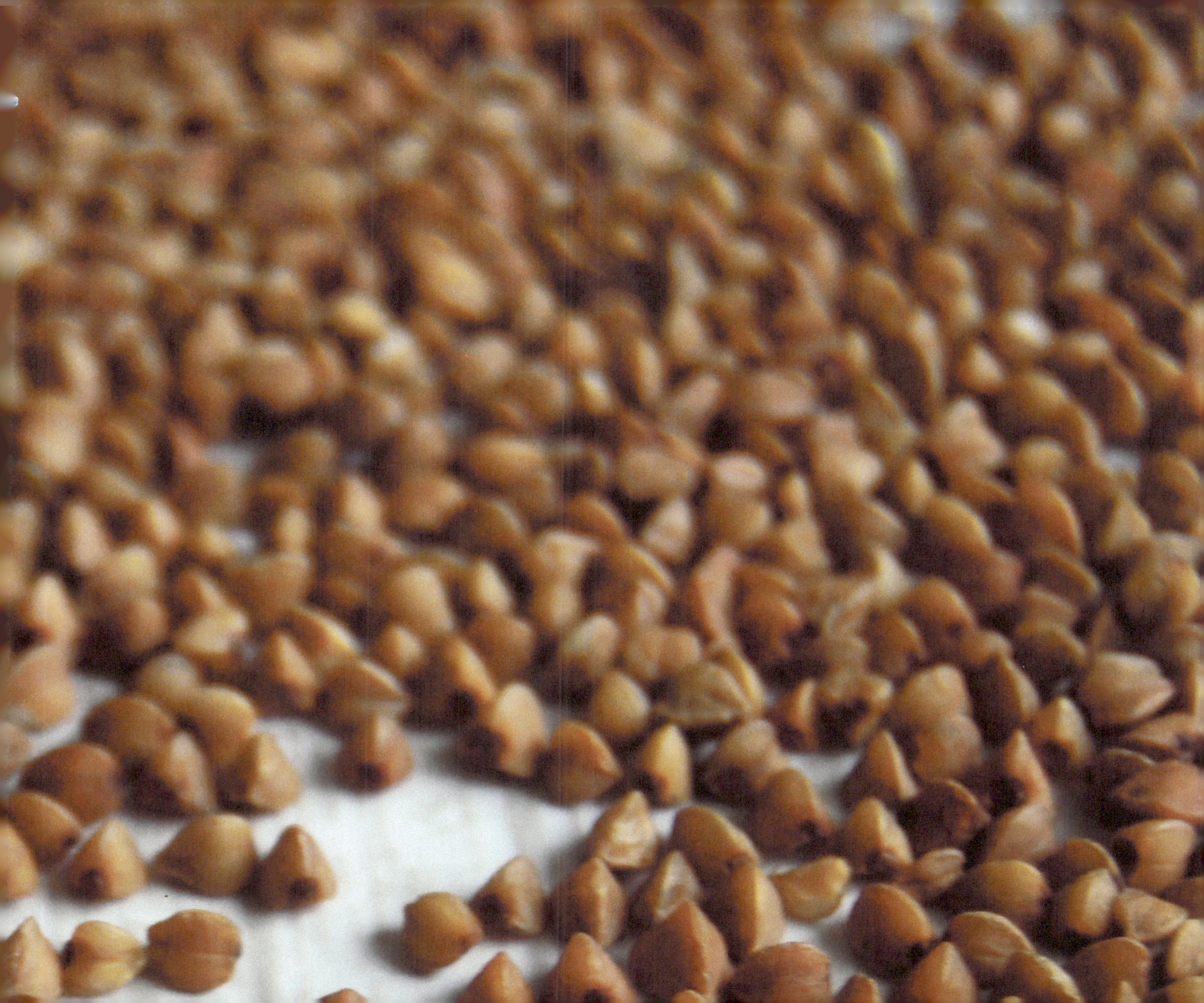

BUTTERCUP SQUASH STUFFED WITH BUCKWHEAT AND BACON

Serve this dish by itself or accompanied by simple salad and meat of your choice.

1 buttercup squash
2 tbsp (30ml) canola oil
1 tsp (5ml) salt
3 tbsp (45ml) butter
1 medium onion, diced
1 cup (250ml) diced double smoked bacon
1 cup (250ml) buckwheat, cooked
¼ cup (60ml) 35% cream
1 cup (250ml) Gruyere cheese, shredded
½ tsp (2.5ml) ground nutmeg
½ tsp (2.5ml) dry thyme

Preheat the oven to 375ºF (200ºC).

Cut the squash into 2 halves. Remove seeds, drizzle with oil, salt and bake at 375ºF (200ºC) oven for about an hour, until flesh becomes tender. Keep it warm in the oven while you work with the filling.

In a medium frying pan heat up butter, add diced onion, bacon, thyme and nutmeg. Cook stirring occasionally for about 4min until bacon becomes translucent. Stir in buckwheat and cream, cook for another 2-3 minutes and set aside. Remove butternut squash from the oven, carefully scrape out the flesh, leaving shells intact. Mix in squash into buckwheat and bacon mix. Refill the squash halves with filling. To up with grated Gruyere cheese. Return to the oven set to broil/grill/ 450ºF (235ºC). Cook for another 15-20 minutes until cheese is well melted.

Serve hot with a slide of light salad and craft beer or Riesling.

Makes 2 large portions

Preparation time: 1 hour 30 minutes

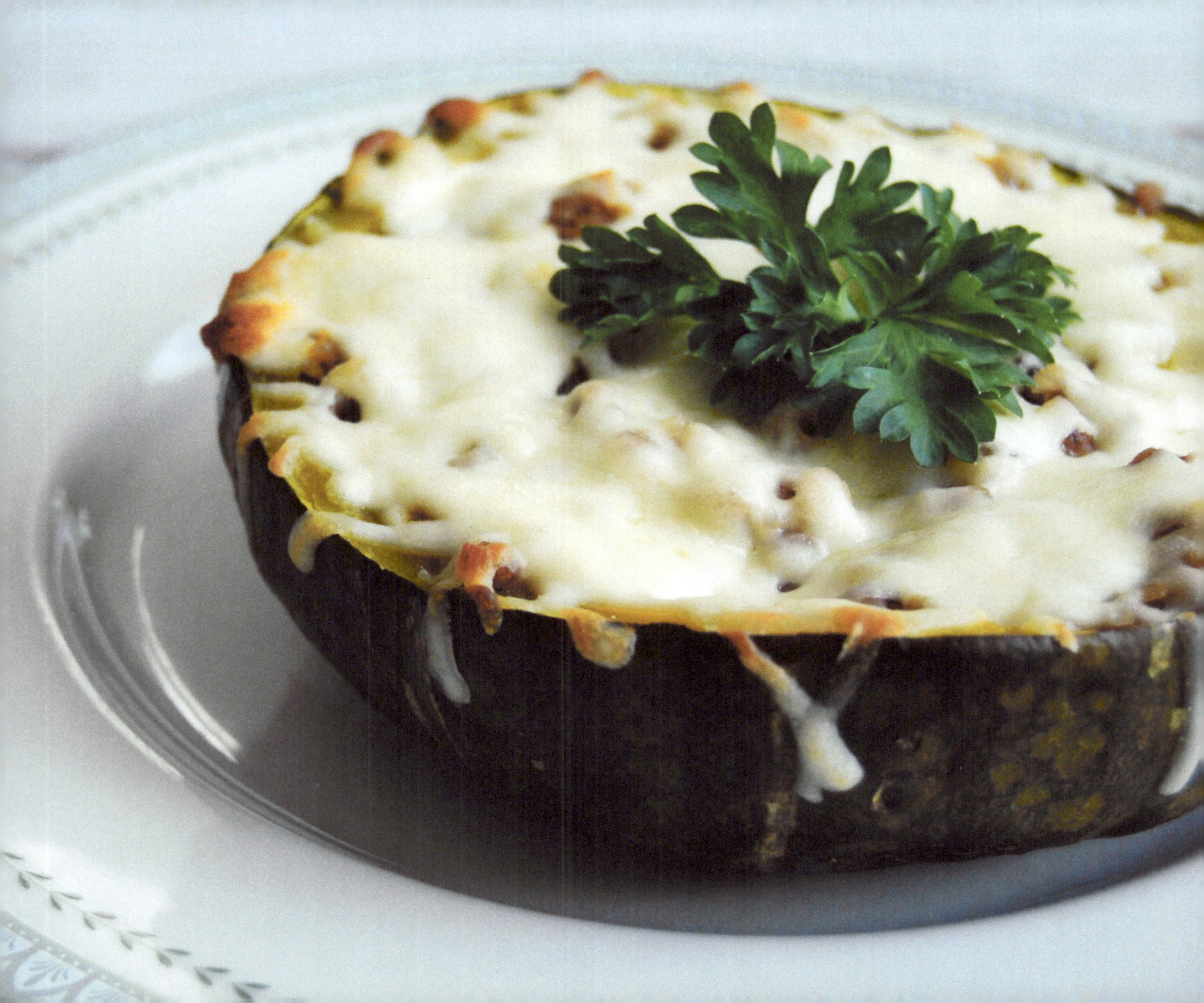

BUCKWHEAT QUICHE LORRAINE

This is my "welcome home" dish that I usually cook when we come back from travelling.
Simple and satisfying, it makes a very easy lunch served along with green salad.

½ cup (125ml) cold butter cubed
1 cup (250ml) wheat all purpose flour
⅔ cup (225ml) buckwheat flour
¼ cup (60ml) water
½ tsp (2.5ml) salt
1 leek stalk cleaned, sliced into thin rounds
1 cup (250ml) double smoked bacon, diced
1 shallot, diced
3 eggs
¼ cup (60ml) 18% cream
½ tbsp (7.5ml) ground black pepper
½ tbsp (7.5ml) nutmeg
½ cup old cheddar cheese

To prepare the dough in a mixing bowl, knead together by hand cold butter, salt, wheat and buckwheat flour. Gradually add about 1/4 cup or less of water to get a dough soft enough to be formed into a ball. Cover with clean kitchen towel and let rest for 30minutes.

Preheat the oven to 200°C (400°F). Grease the pie baking form. Place dough ball between 2 sheets of parchment paper and roll it out into a circle. Line the pie form with the dough, pierce the bottom with a fork in a few places. Place a sheet of parchment paper that was used for rolling out the dough on the top of the dough and fill the tart shell with dry beans. This will ensure the bottom is even without bubbles. Bake for 15 minutes, then remove the baking form from the oven. Reduce oven heat to 180°C (380°F).

To prepare the filling combine in a frying pan sliced leek, bacon and shallot. Heat through and stir-fry for about 3-5 minutes on medium heat until bacon becomes slightly transparent. In a bowl, whisk together eggs, cream, black pepper and nutmeg. Place the leek and bacon mix on the bottom of the tart shell, pour over the egg mixture, sprinkle with cheese on top.

Place in the oven and bake for about 25-30 minutes until egg filling solidifies and cheese lightly browns a bit.

Slice and serve hot with a side of light salad and a glass of cider or Riesling to accompany.

Makes 1 quiche

Preparation time: 1 hour

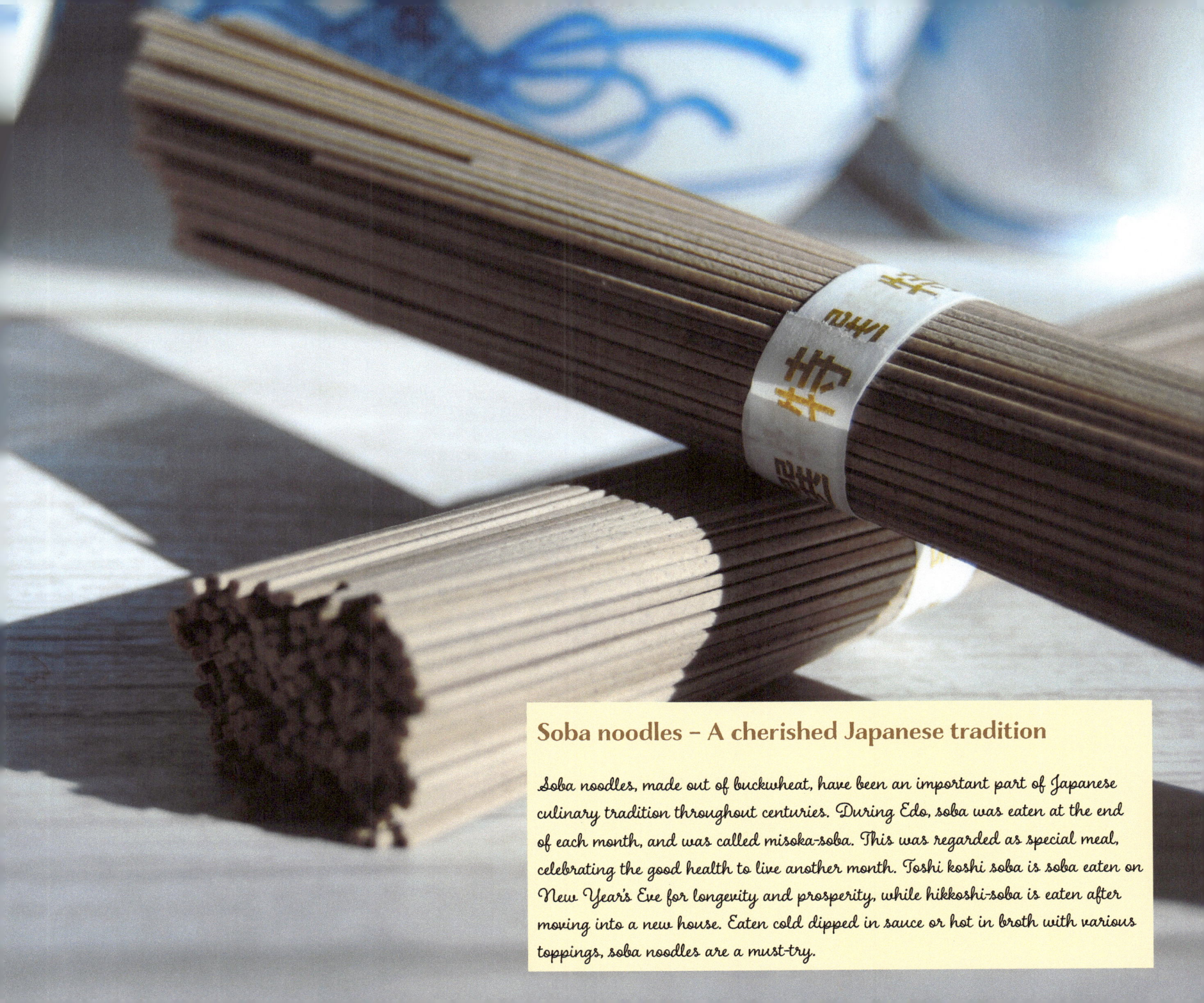

Soba noodles – A cherished Japanese tradition

Soba noodles, made out of buckwheat, have been an important part of Japanese culinary tradition throughout centuries. During Edo, soba was eaten at the end of each month, and was called misoka-soba. This was regarded as special meal, celebrating the good health to live another month. Toshi koshi soba is soba eaten on New Year's Eve for longevity and prosperity, while hikkoshi-soba is eaten after moving into a new house. Eaten cold dipped in sauce or hot in broth with various toppings, soba noodles are a must-try.

TOSHI KOSHI SOBA

Ready to ring in the New Year? Make sure this toshi koshi soba is on your New Year's Eve menu.

1.5 L bonito or kombu dashi stock
⅔ cup (225ml) soy sauce
¼ cup + 2 tbsp (90ml) mirin
1 tbsp (15ml) sugar
1 cup + 2 tbsp (280ml) tsuyu (optional)
200g soba buckwheat noodles (about 2 bundles)
2 spring onions
2 tbsp (30ml) tempura flakes
4 large shrimp, cooked
2 tbsp (30ml) wakame flakes
2 sprigs of cilantro
2 slices kamaboko fish cake (optional)

Kombu dashi stock

You can make home-made kombu dashi stock by soaking kombu seaweed in 1L of water overnight. Then heat it until small bubbles appear. Do not boil the seaweed. Remove it from ready to boil water and add 3 cups (30g) of bonito flakes and let simmer for 1 minute. Turn off the heat and let it sit for 10 minutes. Strain dashi stock and use it as a soup base.

Makes 2 servings

Preparation time: 20 minutes

To prepare the bonito or kombu dashi broth follow the instructions on the packet or see home made kombu dashi stock recipe.

In a large pot, add the mirin to the dashi stock and simmer gently for a few minutes. Now, add the sugar and let it dissolve before adding the soy sauce.

In separate pot, bring 1L of water to the boil. Add the soba noodles, reduce the heat to a simmer and cook for about 5 minutes until tender. Drain the noodles and rinse them in cold water. Next, thinly slice the spring onions and cilantro.

Pour warm broth into serving bowls, then add the noodles and garnish with your spring onions, tempura flakes, wakame, shrimp and cilantro. Use fish cake slices for garnish as well if you have them available.

Note: if you are short on time, replace the soy sauce, mirin and sugar with tsuyu sauce. Just use a ratio of 1 part tsuyu to 5 parts dashi stock when making your soba noodle broth.

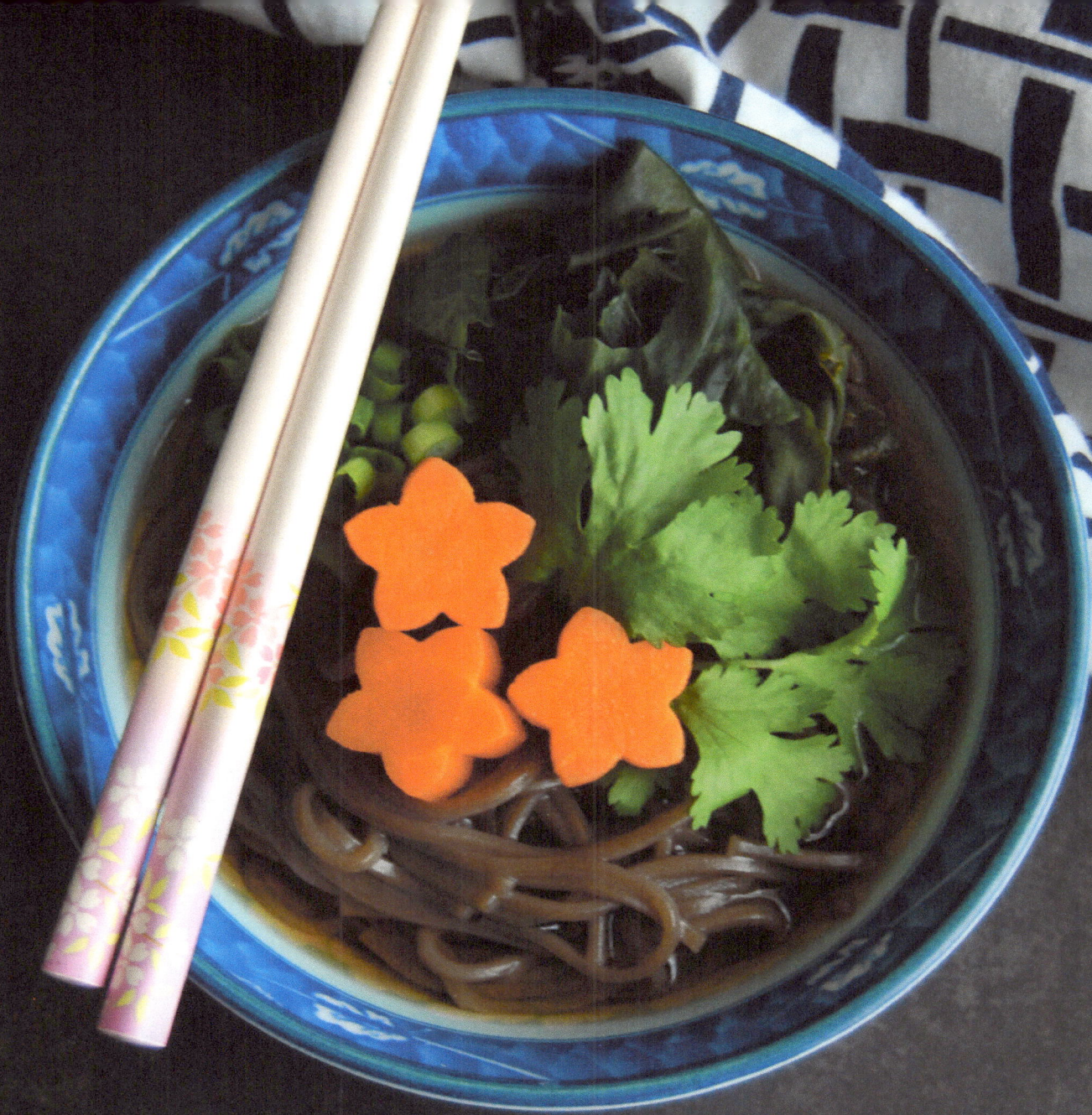

BUCKWHEAT HALUSHKI WITH SMOKED PORK BACK FAT AND SHALLOTS

Halushki is a traditional Ukrainian dish that can be made from different kinds of flour. Buckwheat halushki have a particular earthy nutty flavour.

2 cups (500ml) buckwheat flour
½ cups + 1 ½ cups (125ml + 375ml) water
2 eggs
3 shallots
0.5 lb (200g) pork back fat smoked and salted

In a deep skillet, sautee diced pork back fat with diced shallots until golden, then separate into two portions, reserve one for later, the other portion place into a saucepan, add 3 cups of water and bring to rolling boil.

Combine buckwheat flour, ½ cup water, eggs and mix into soft dough. Roll it out to about ¼ in (0.5 cm) and cut into bite-size square pieces. Drop the dough into boiling back fat and shallot broth, cook for about 20 min. until they float up on the surface. Remove from broth with perforated spoon and place into a serving bowl. Serve hot halushki as soon as possible with the broth that they been cooking in, served in a separate bowl.

Makes 4 servings

Preparation time: 30 minutes

BELL PEPPERS STUFFED WITH BUCKWHEAT AND BEEF

Full of colour and flavour these peppers freeze well. Perfect idea for work or school lunch where you can re-heat this dish in the middle of the day.

4 bell peppers of your preferred colour
1 cup (250ml) buckwheat
1 tbsp (15ml) butter
1 cup (250ml) ground beef
1 shallot, diced
1 tbsp (15ml) ground black pepper
½ cup (125ml) shredded carrot
1 tsp (5ml) salt
1 tsp (5ml) oregano

Cut off tops with stem from the bell peppers, carefully remove seeds, keep the lids and arrange bottoms of the peppers in a ceramic deep oven proof dish, so that they sit quite tight.

Cook the buckwheat as described in simple buckwheat recipe on p. – 31

In a frying pan, combine butter, beef, shallot, black pepper, shredded carrot, salt and mayoram. Stir fry it for about 3-4 min., then add this mixture to the cooked buckwheat and stir well. Fill the bottoms of bell peppers with filling, pressing the filling in with a spoon to make sure all crevices are filled. Cover with tops and bake at 180°C (360°F) for about 25-30 minutes until bell peppers are tender and filling is cooked through.

Serve hot with a dollop of sour cream and some fresh parsley.

Makes 4 servings

Preparation time 1 hour

BEEF AND ROOT VEGETABLE STEW WITH BUCKWHEAT

Cooking it nice and slow fills the house with fantastic aroma. Perfect for cold end of winter days.

3 lb (1.3kg) beef chuck roasts
4 tsp (20ml) olive oil
1 cup (250ml) white wine
2 medium carrots, chopped into thick rounds, peeled
1 medium parsnip, chopped into thick rounds, peeled
1 cup (250ml) leeks, sliced into rounds
1 tsp (5ml) cumin
1 tsp (5ml) ground turmeric
1 tsp (5ml) ground cinnamon
1 tsp (5ml) ginger
1 tsp (5ml) salt
1 tsp (5ml) ground black pepper
500ml can diced tomatoes
1 lb (500g) sweet potato, peeled, diced into large cubes
2 cups (500ml) buckwheat

Trim and discard visible fat from the beef, and cut it into 1-inch cubes. In a large skillet over medium-high heat, heat the oil. Place several beef pieces in the frying pan and brown evenly from all sides, move them into a heavy cast iron pot. Work in batches until all beef is evenly browned. Add 1 cup of white wine to the frying pan and scrape up the browned bits. Add this liquid to the pot with beef. Add the carrots, parsnip, leek leaves, cumin, turmeric, cinnamon, ginger, salt, pepper, brown sugar, and tomatoes to the pot. Distribute the partially cooked beef in a single layer on top of the vegetables. Top with sweet potatoes, cover and bake at 180°C (360°F) for about 3 hours. The stew is ready to serve when the sweet potatoes are tender when pierced with a fork.

In a large skillet, roast the buckwheat as described i simple buckwheat recipe on p.31. Move the roasted buckwheat to a large saucepan. Cover with 4 cups cold water and cook for about 20 minutes on medium low heat, until grains are tender.

To serve spoon some buckwheat into a deep bowl, top with beef stew. Serve hot.

Makes 4 servings

Preparation time: 3 hours 20 minutes

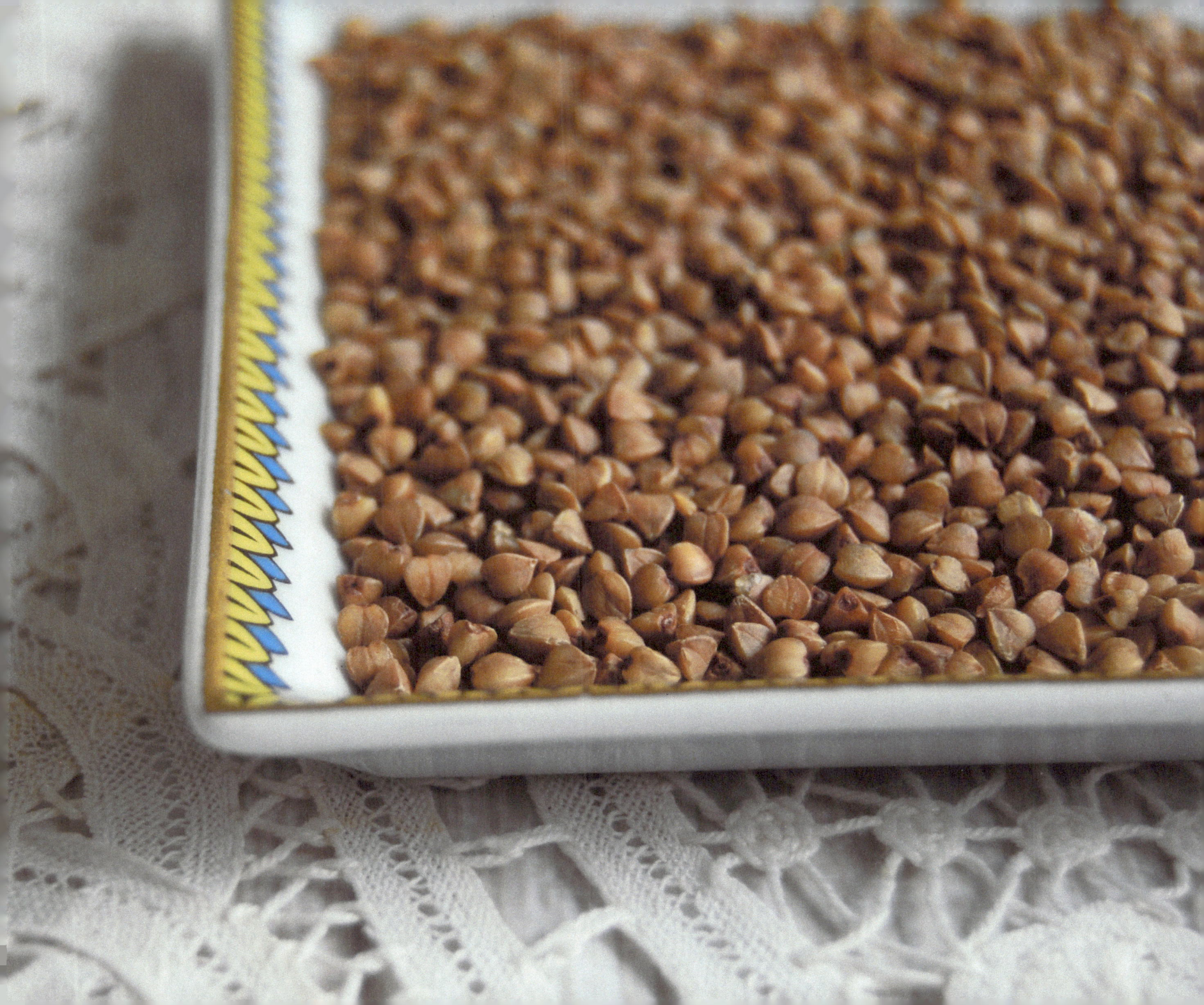

PORK CHOPS WITH BUCKWHEAT
AND TRUFFLE OIL

Dinner made simple. Add your favourite dried herbs to the frying pan to season the pork to your liking.

1 tsp (5ml) herbes de Provence
2 thick pork shoulder chops
1 cup (250ml) buckwheat, roasted
2 shallots, thinly sliced
2 tbsp (30ml) butter
1 tsp (5ml) truffle oil
½ tsp (2.5ml) salt
½ tsp (2.5ml) fresh ground black pepper

Heat vegetable oil in a large heavy skillet over high. Add herbes des Provence to the frying pan and stir. Season pork with salt and cook until browned but still pink in the center, about 4 minutes per side. Add 1 Tbsp. butter and spoon melted butter over chops, turning them once, then continue cooking for another 1-2 min. Transfer meat to a cutting board and let rest 10 minutes. In a medium saucepan cook buckwheat in 2 cups water until tender.

In a small frying, pan melt butter, stir fry shallots until lightly golden (for about 5 minutes). Stir the shallots into the cooked buckwheat, season with truffle oil, salt and pepper and spoon into serving bowls. Slice the meat and serve on the side with the buckwheat.

Makes 2 servings

Preparation time: 30 minutes

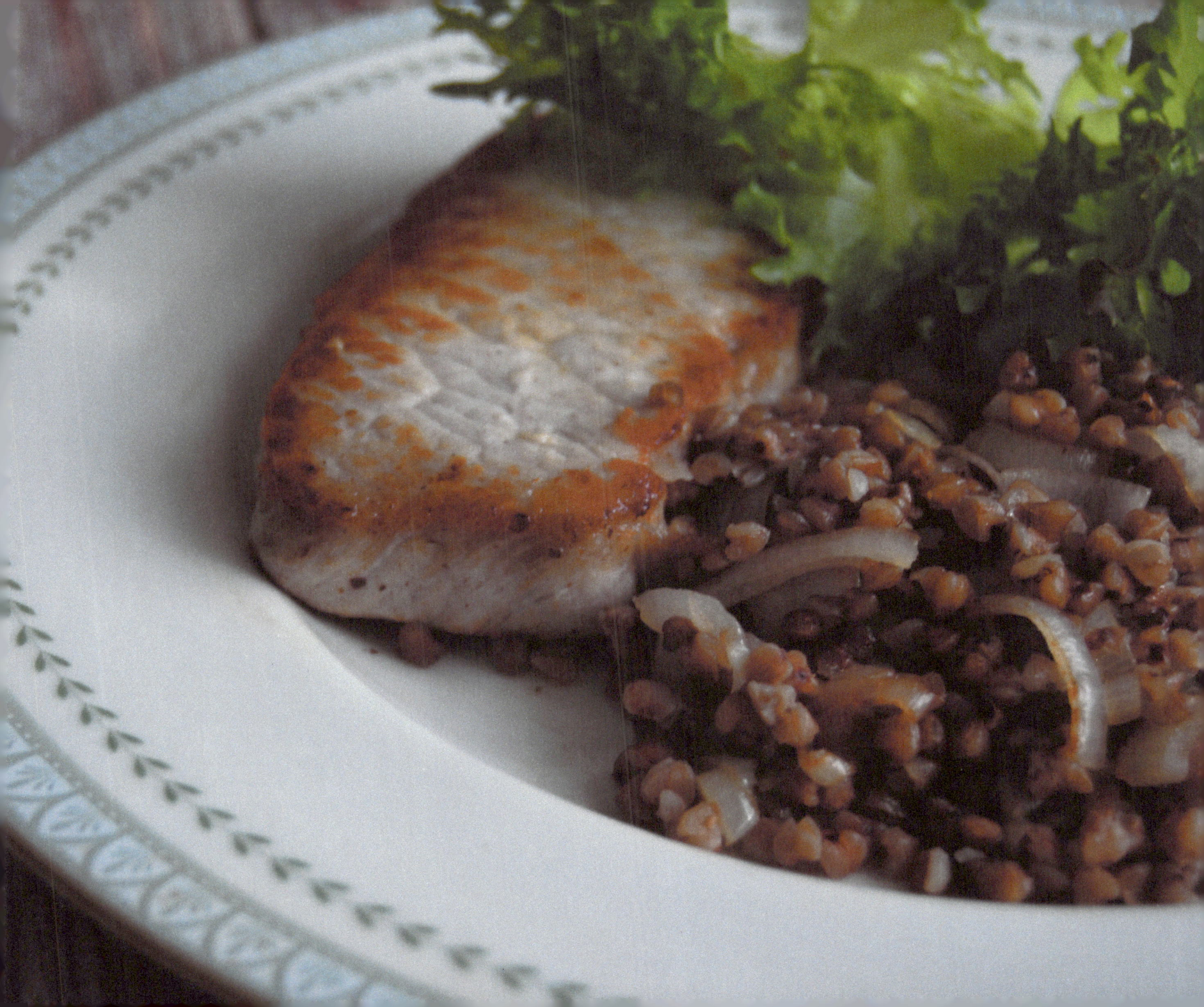

CREPE BRETONNES WITH HAM AND EGG

This recipe I encountered for the first time in the town of corsairs - Saint Malo, France. Salty breeze and romantic atmosphere of a French pirate bay generously compliments this dish. To re-create the atmosphere serve these crepes along with fresh salad and cider, preferably out in the fresh air.

2 cups buckwheat flour
4 eggs
½ tsp salt
Water
4 slices smoked ham
4 eggs
1 tsp salt
1 tsp ground black pepper
4 tbsp shredded Gruyere cheese

In a mixing bowl combine buckwheat flour, eggs, salt and mix well making sure there are no lumps. Gradually add just enough water to get a thick smooth batter. Let it rest, covered with a clean tea towel for about 15-20 minutes at room temperature.

Slightly grease crepe maker or shallow frying pan. Stir the batter, add a bit of water if it thickens up too much. With a ladle spread the batter onto tilted crepe maker into a layer as thin as possible, making sure it covers evenly the entire surface. Bake at medium-high heat from one side and flip over to another. Transfer the galette into a plate and keep it warm in the oven, set at minimal heat, while you work on the next galette. Continue until all batter is used up.

To serve place the galette on the crepe maker or frying pan on low heat, place slice of ham in the middle, break one egg and let it heat until egg starts to solidify. Season with salt and pepper and fold in the galette form 4 sides inwards like an envelope, leaving the egg yolk exposed. Spread some shredded Gruyere cheese on top and gently slide the galette into the serving plate and serve immediately.

Makes approximately 4 large galettes

Preparation time: 20 minutes

BUCKWHEAT MEXICAN BOWL

Great idea for a satisfying summer lunch. Goes well with a refreshing cold beer and perhaps a palm tree and a pool side.

2 cups (500ml) buckwheat, raw
1 large avocado, diced
⅓ cup (75ml) corn kernels, canned
¼ cup (60ml) red onion, diced
2 medium tomato, diced
1 medium green pepper, diced
½ cup (125ml) fresh cilantro, chopped
¼ cup (60ml) fresh lime juice
4 tbsp (60ml) olive oil
2 tsp (10ml) chili flakes

In a small saucepan cook buckwheat in 4 cups of water as described in simple buckwheat recipe on p. 31. Cool to room temperature. In a large bowl combine buckwheat, avocado, corn, onion, tomato, green bell pepper and mix well all ingredients. Spoon the mixture into serving bowls, dress with fresh chopped cilantro, lime juice, olive oil and some chili flakes.

Makes 4 servings

Preparation time: 30 minutes

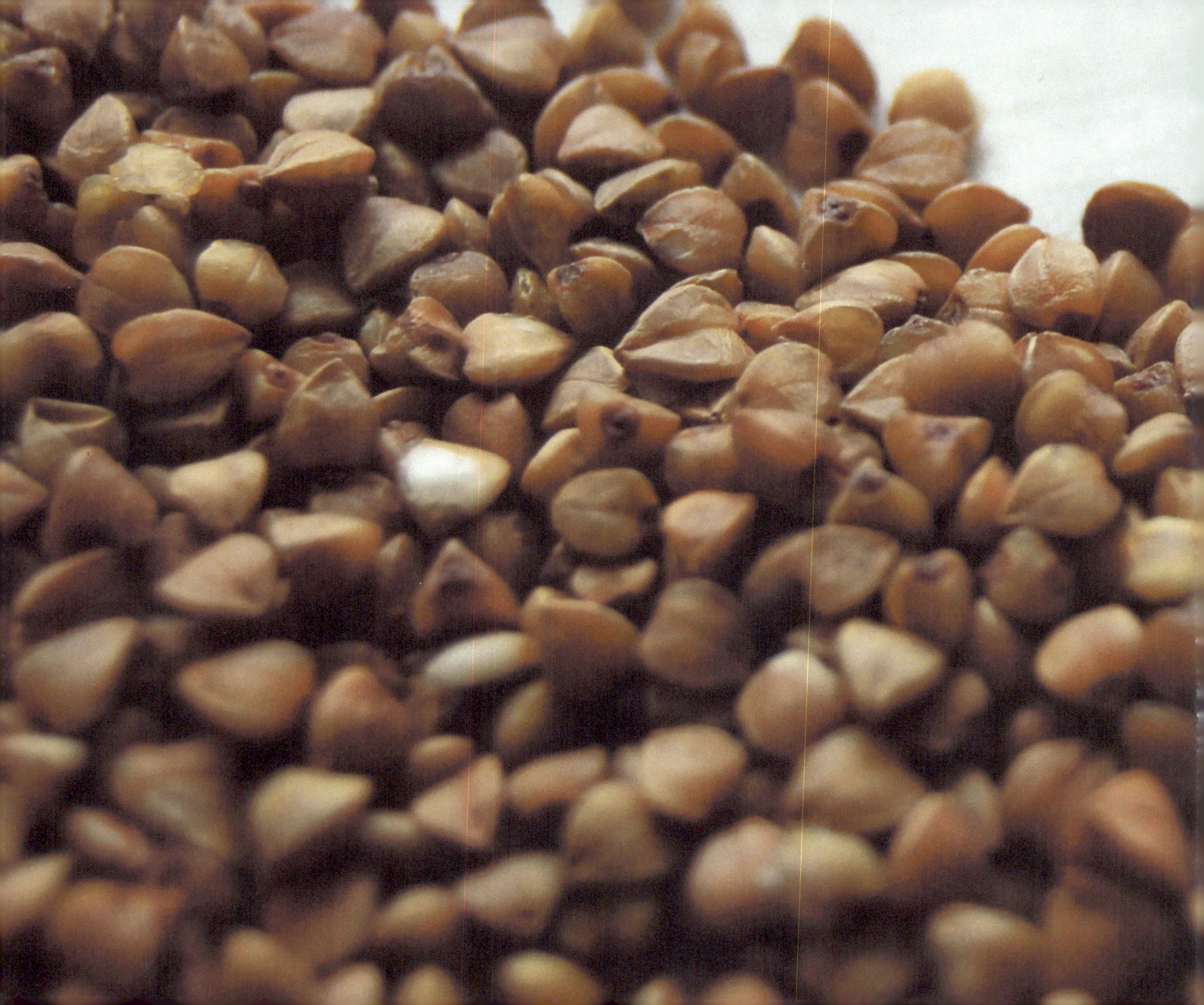

DESSERTS

From dainty to rustic, full of silky cream and amber honey these desserts will captivate you.

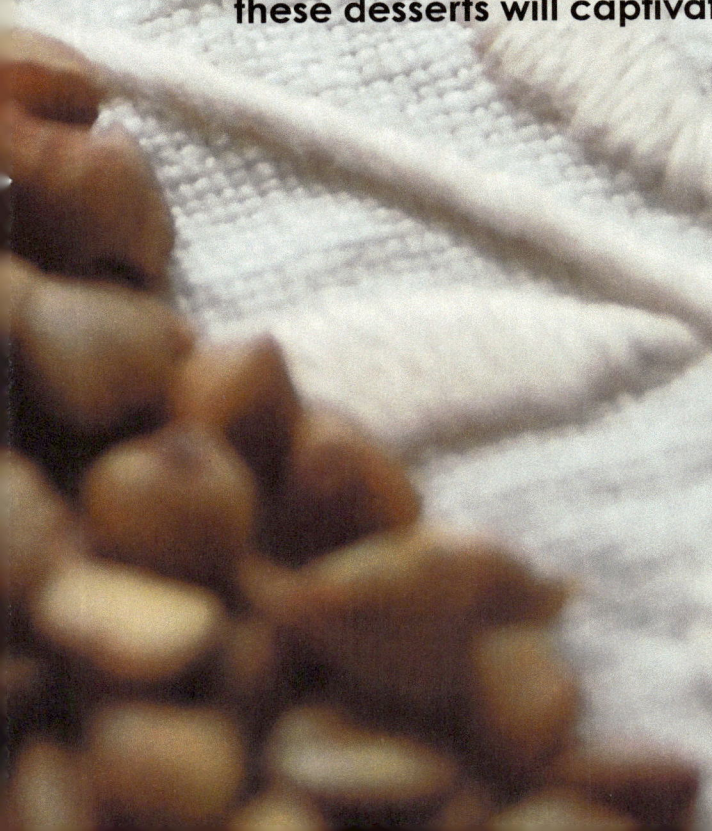

SWEET COCONUT MILK AND BUCKWHEAT PORRIDGE WITH STRAWBERRIES

Freshness of strawberries really stands out in this smooth porridge. Great as a summer breakfast.

1 L coconut milk
2 cups (500ml) uncooked buckwheat
3 tbsp (45ml) sugar
2 tbsp (30ml) butter
½ tsp (2.5ml) coconut extract
½ tsp (2.5ml) salt
1 cup (250ml) small size fresh strawberries

Makes 4 servings

Preparation time: 45 minutes

Cover buckwheat with coconut milk and simmer on medium-low heat until buckwheat is fully cooked and tender, about 15-20 minutes. Remove buckwheat from heat; stir in 2 tablespoons sugar, coconut extract, salt and butter. Finely dice ½ cup of strawberries and stir into the porridge. Use the rest of the strawberries as a topping to decorate the bowls of porridge before serving.

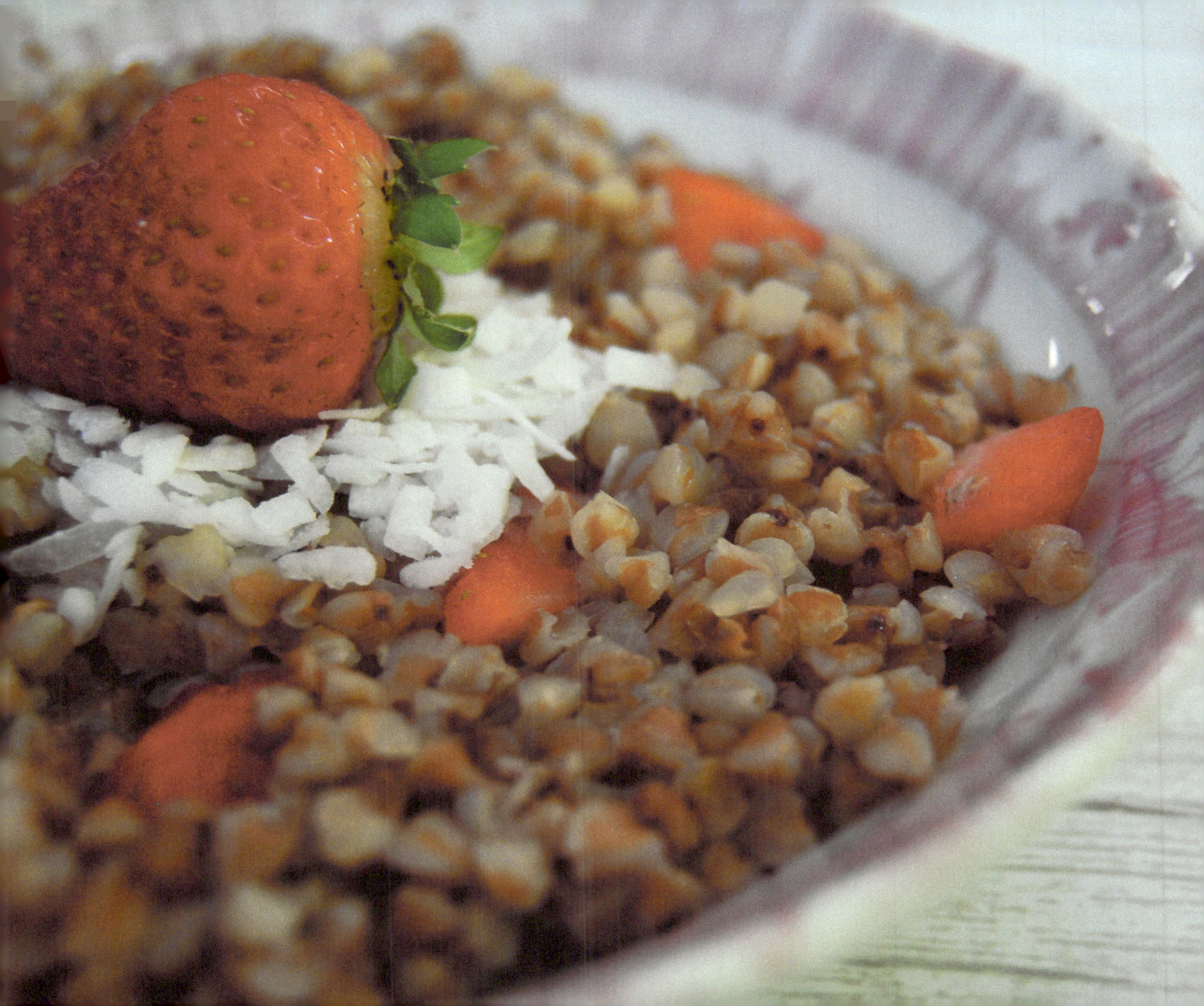

BUCKWHEAT BREAKFAST PANCAKES
WITH BLUEBERRY SYRUP

Have the kids do all the prep and dress their own pancakes.

1 cup (250ml) buckwheat flour
⅓ cup (75ml) all purpose wheat flour
1 ½ tsp (7.5ml) baking powder
½ tsp (2.5ml) salt
1 tbsp (15ml) sugar
½ tsp (2.5ml) vanilla extract
1 tbsp (15ml) vegetable oil
1 ⅔ cup (475ml) water or milk or almond milk
½ cup (125ml) blueberries
¼ cup (60ml) sugar

In a mixing bowl combine buckwheat flour, wheat flour, baking powder, salt, sugar and vanilla extract. Mix well. While mixing the dry ingredients add vegetable oil and water and mix everything together. Pre-heat non stick frying pan and spoon the batter to form pancakes. Cook from both sides on medium heat until surface has a nice lightly golden colour.

To prepare the syrup in a small saucepan combine blueberries and a ¼ cup of sugar and heat while stirring once in a while for about 5 minutes so that berries give off juice and sugar is completely melted. Serve hot pancakes with some syrup drizzled over them or on the side.

Makes 6 servings

Preparation time: 25 minutes

BUCKWHEAT WAFFLES WITH MAPLE SYRUP CREAM SAUCE

Great breakfast for early spring while maple syrup is at its best.

1 cup (250ml) buckwheat flour
⅓ cup (75ml) all purpose wheat flour
1 ½ tsp (7.5ml) baking powder
½ tsp (2.5ml) salt
1 tbsp (15ml) sugar
½ tsp (2.5ml) vanilla extract
1 tbsp (15ml) vegetable oil
1 ⅔ cup (475ml) water or milk or almond milk
½ cup (125ml) 35% cream
2 tbsp (30ml) maple syrup

In a mixing bowl, combine buckwheat flour, wheat flour, baking powder, salt, sugar and vanilla extract. Mix well. While mixing the dry ingredients, add vegetable oil and water and mix everything together. Pre-heat your waffle maker and cook waffles according to the waffle maker instructions.

To prepare the cream sauce, place cream into a medium bowl and gently whisk in the maple syrup to obtain smooth runny texture. For best results use cream directly from refrigerator. Serve the hot waffles with the maple cream sauce.

Makes approximately 4 servings

Preparation time: 25 minutes

BUCKWHEAT CREPES WITH APPLE COMPOTE AND BUCKWHEAT HONEY

The first time I tried a galette de sarrasin (buckwheat crepe), it was in Saint Malo, France, fortress city known to be a corsair haven. Here is my version of this corsair dessert.

1 ¼ cups (310ml) buckwheat flour
4 large eggs
¼ cup (60ml) vegetable oil plus additional for skillet
1 cup (250ml) 2% milk
1 cup (250ml) (or more) water
¼ tsp (60ml) salt
2 cups (500ml) tart apples, peeled, diced
2 tbsp (30ml) sugar
1 tbsp (15ml) butter
2 tbsp (30ml) water
½ tsp (2.5ml) cinnamon
⅓ cup (75ml) buckwheat honey

Place flour, eggs, oil, milk and water into a blender and blend to obtain smooth runny batter. Heat a medium size crepe pan or frying pan or skillet (non stick) over medium-high heat. Add about 1 tsp oil and a 1/3 cup of batter to the skillet (best use a soup ladle to measure out equal amounts of batter per each crepe); tilt to evenly coat the entire surface of the frying pan. Cook crepe until golden on the bottom, adjusting heat to prevent burning, 30 to 45 seconds. Using spatula, turn crepe over, cook for 30 seconds and transfer to plate. Repeat with remaining batter, stacking the crepes on a big plate.

To prepare apple compote in a small sauce pan heat up the apples with sugar, butter, water and cinnamon on low heat, constantly stirring. Cook the apples for about 10-15 minutes until tender but not too soft. To serve, place a few tablespoons of apple compote in the middle of the crepe, fold crepe edges from 4 sides towards the middle like an envelope and drizzle generously with buckwheat honey before serving.

Makes approximately 4 large crepes

Preparation time: 30 minutes

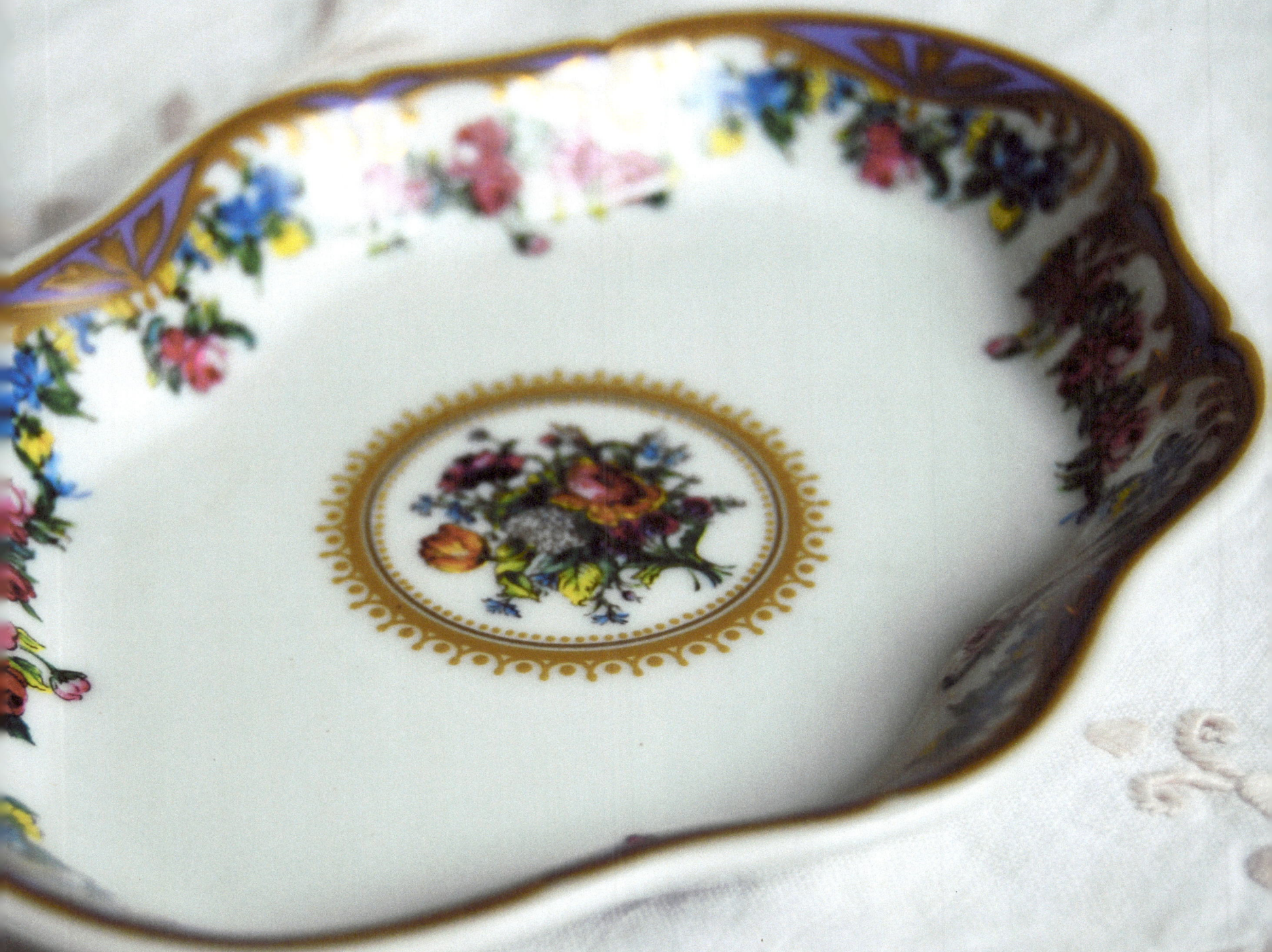

BREAKFAST BUCKWHEAT PORRIDGE WITH CARDAMOM PEARS AND ALMONDS

Loaded with flavour, it makes a great breakfast or a fantastic work lunch as it can easily be packed into a thermos.

1L whole milk
2 cups (500ml) uncooked buckwheat
2 tbsp plus 2 tsp (30ml + 10ml) sugar, divided
2 tbsp (30ml) butter divided
½ tsp (2.5ml) vanilla extract
¼ tsp (1.5ml) almond extract
¼ tsp (1.5ml) salt
1 tbsp (15ml) butter
1 cup (250ml) chopped ripe pear
2 tbsp (30ml) water
½ tsp (2.5ml) ground cardamom
¼ cup (60ml) sliced almonds, toasted

Makes 4 servings

Preparation time: 45 minutes

Cover buckwheat with milk and simmer on medium-low heat until buckwheat is fully cooked and tender, about 15-20 minutes. Remove buckwheat from heat; stir in 2 tablespoons sugar, butter, vanilla, almond extract, salt.

Heat a small non stick frying pan over medium-high heat. Melt butter and add pear, remaining 2 teaspoons sugar, 2 tablespoons water, and cardamom to pan. Bring to a simmer; cover and cook about 3-4 minutes. Remove from heat. Spoon cereal evenly into 4 bowls. Top evenly with pear mixture and almonds.

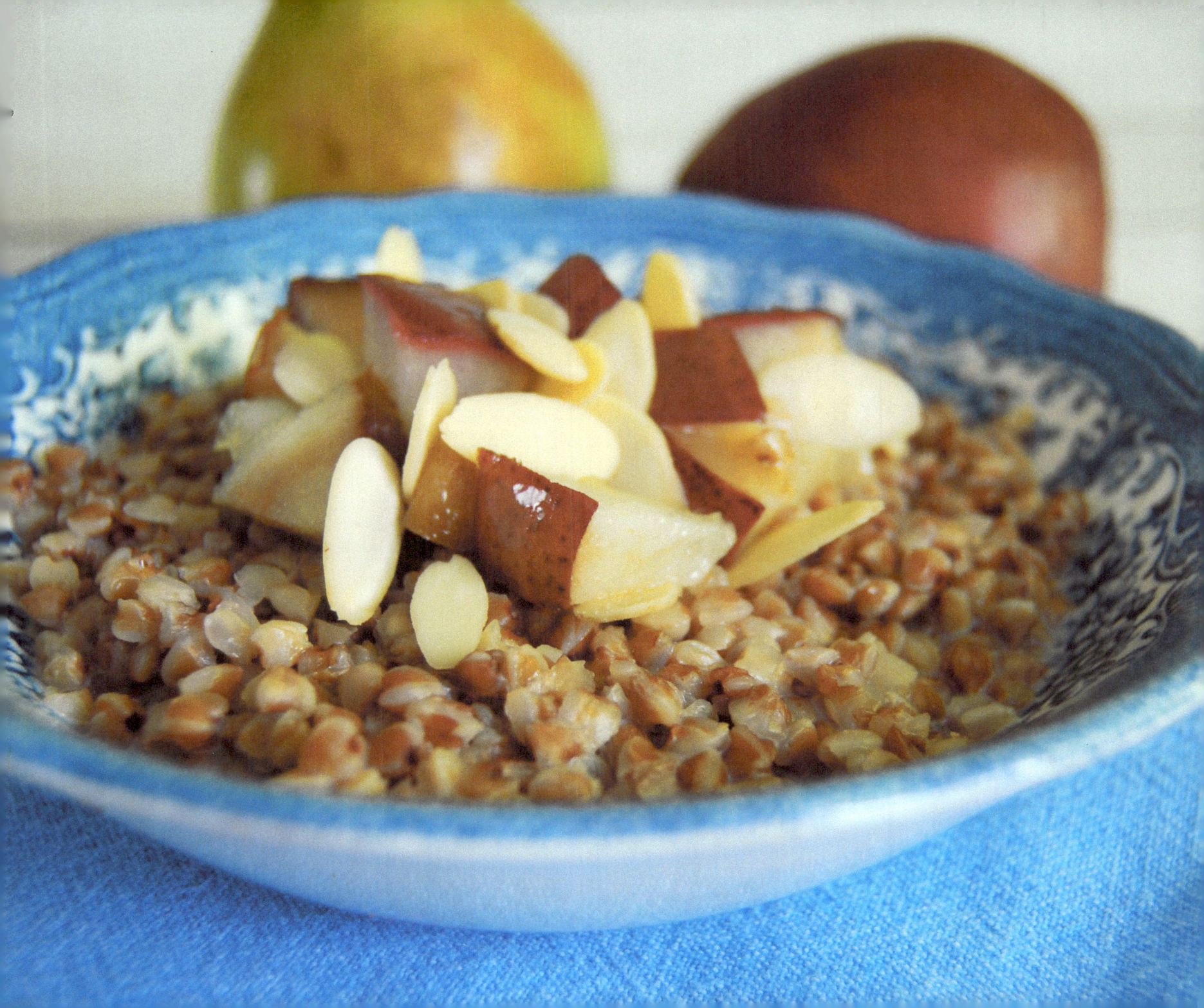

BUCKWHEAT AND CHOCOLATE SOUFFLÉ WITH FLEUR D'ORANGE WHIPPED CREAM

Kids love this dessert. Earthy nutty flavour of the soufflé goes well with the floral light whipped cream topping. Perfect for a dainty tea party or a kid's birthday.

½ cup (125ml) buckwheat
1¼ cup (310ml) milk
½ tsp (2.5ml) vanilla extract
½ tsp (2.5ml) salt
4 tbsp (60ml) sugar
2 egg whites
2 tsp (10ml) cocoa powder
1 tsp (5ml) corn starch
2 egg whites
½ cup (125ml) 35% whipping cream
½ tsp (2.5ml) fleur d'orange water
1 tbsp (15ml) sugar

Makes 4 small servings or 2 large ones

Preparation time: 40 minutes

In a medium saucepan combine buckwheat, 1 cup milk, vanilla extract, salt and sugar and cook buckwheat on medium heat until soft – about 20 minutes. In a blender, combine cocoa, corn starch, buckwheat ¼ cup milk and puree in a blender to get smooth texture. In a separate bowl, beat the egg whites into stiff peaks and fold carefully into the buckwheat mix. Take ceramic ramekins and carefully grease the interior with a small piece of butter. Spread the batter into the ramekins, filling them to 2/3. Bake at 200ºC (375ºF) for 20-25 minutes.

In a separate bowl, whip together whipping cream (preferably cold as it will whip up better and faster), the fleur d'orange water and sugar. Spoon or pipe out the whipped cream on top of soufflé just before serving.

Fleur d'orange water can be found in bakery isle in some grocery stores and in ethnic stores that carry middle eastern products. In case you can not find it you can use fleur d'orange extract (keep in mind it has a completely different floral aroma from orange fruit extract).

BUCKWHEAT COOKIES

Light and nutty, they will make a great addition to your Christmas baking. Go perfectly well with a cup of tea or coffee.

1 cup (250ml) buckwheat flour
1 cup (250ml) wheat flour
2 eggs
2 tbsp (30ml) buckwheat honey
½ cup (125ml) sugar
1 tsp (5ml) vanilla extract
¾ cup (180ml) butter softened
1 tsp (5ml) baking powder

Makes about 12 cookies

Preparation time: 30 minutes

Preheat the oven to 180°C (360°F).

In a bowl, combine buckwheat and wheat flour, eggs, buckwheat honey, sugar, vanilla extract, butter and baking powder. If dough turns out a bit too runny, add a bit more of wheat flour. Dough should be thick enough so you could roll it into small balls. Form balls about size of a cherry, place them onto a baking tray lined with parchment paper. Bake at 180°C (360°F) for about 15-20 minutes until toothpick inserted in the middle comes out dry. Let the cookies cool down before moving them into a serving bowl.

If honey is crystallized, it did not go bad. It is still perfectly good for use. In order to liquefy crystallized honey, place the honey into a small saucepan, place that pan on top of a larger one ¼ filled with water. Place this tower onto small-medium heat and stir constantly. As soon as all crystals melt and honey becomes smooth and liquid again – remove from heat and transfer into a glass jar.

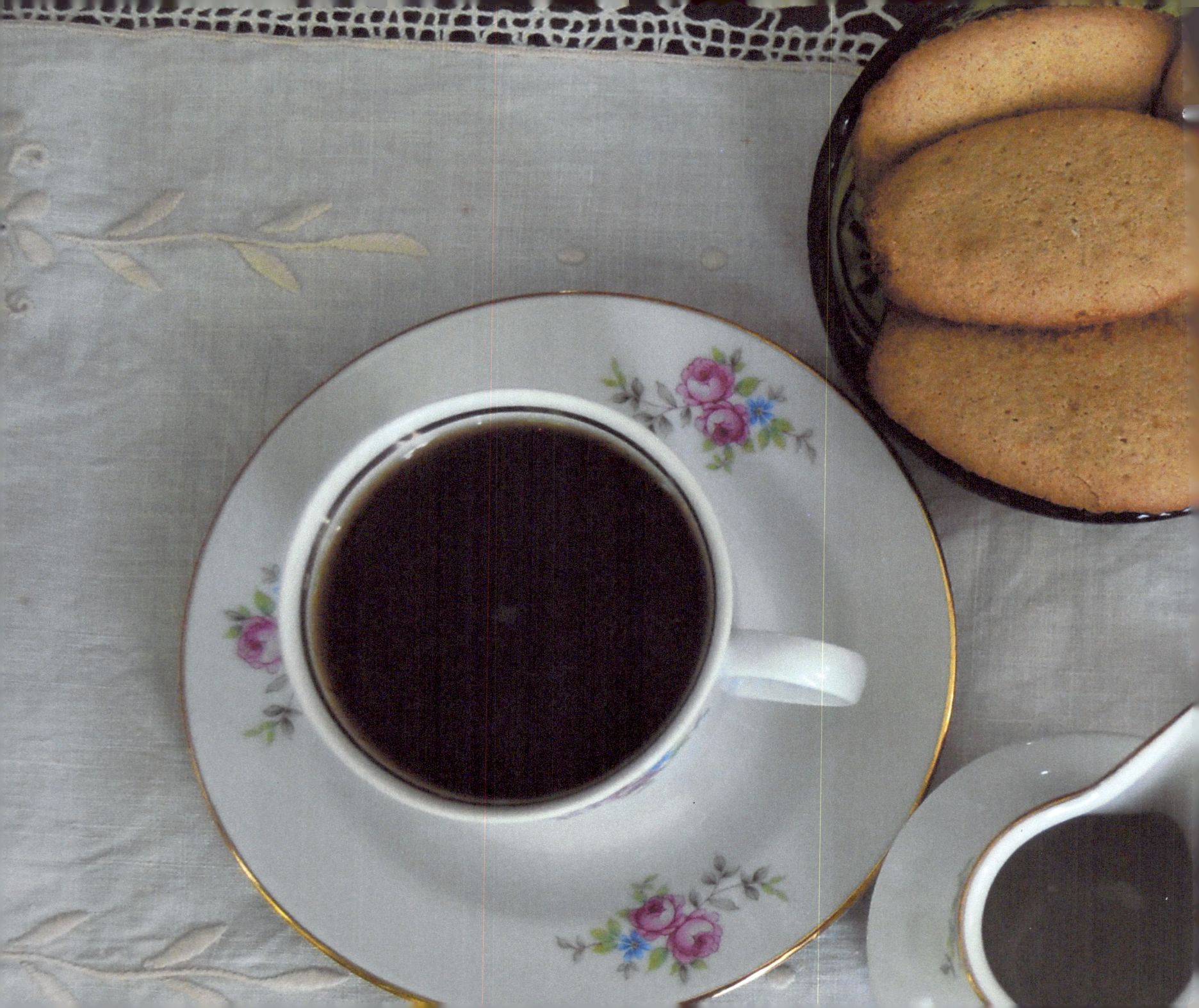

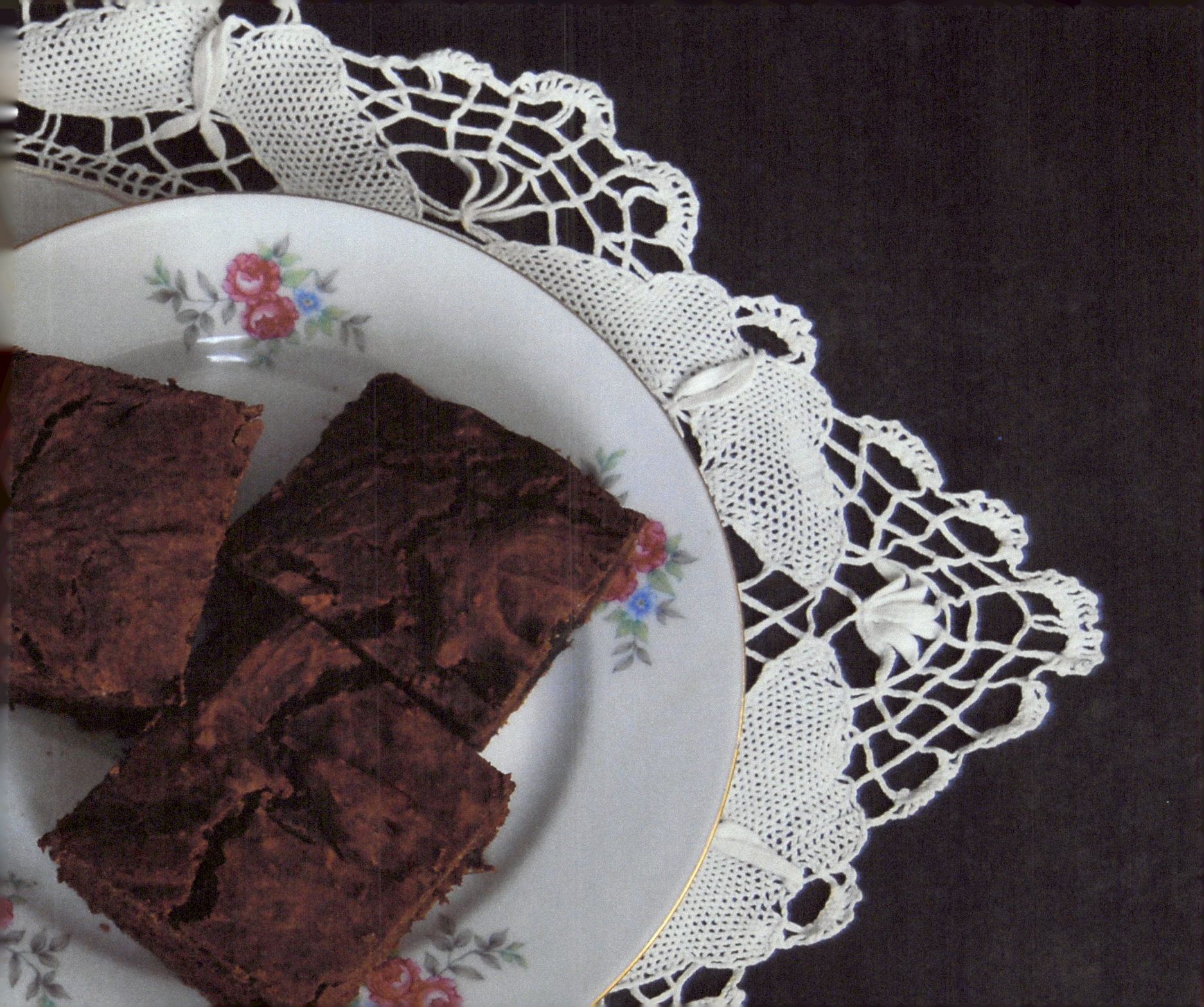

BUCKWHEAT ALMOND
AND NECTARINE CAKE

Be it tea party or birthday party, any kind of celebration deserves this kind of cake.

5 eggs
1 cup (250ml) sugar
½ cup (125ml) butter softened
1 cup (250ml) ground almonds
1 cup (250ml) buckwheat flour
4 nectarines, pits removed, diced
1 tsp (5ml) baking powder
½ tsp (2.5ml) ground cinnamon
½ tsp (2.5ml) nutmeg

Makes 1 cake

Preparation time: 1 hour

In a mixing bowl, whisk together (or use a hand mixer) eggs with sugar until smooth thick foam forms. Preheat the oven to 200ºC (375ºF). Carefully whisk in the buckwheat flour, baking powder, cinnamon and nutmeg. Carefully fold the nectarines into the dough and pour the dough into round spring cake form that has been greased and sprinkled with a little bit of buckwheat flour. Bake in preheated oven for about 30-35 minutes until knife inserted in the middle comes out dry and top crust is nicely golden.

Remove cake from the form, place on serving plate and dust with a little bit for powdered sugar for decoration.

Cake fillings – feel free to replace nectarines with any dense fruit of your choice – pineapple, apples, pears, plums work great. So do berries – cranberries, blueberries. Fresh or frozen they are equally great in this cake. Try to use seasonal fruit as much as possible.

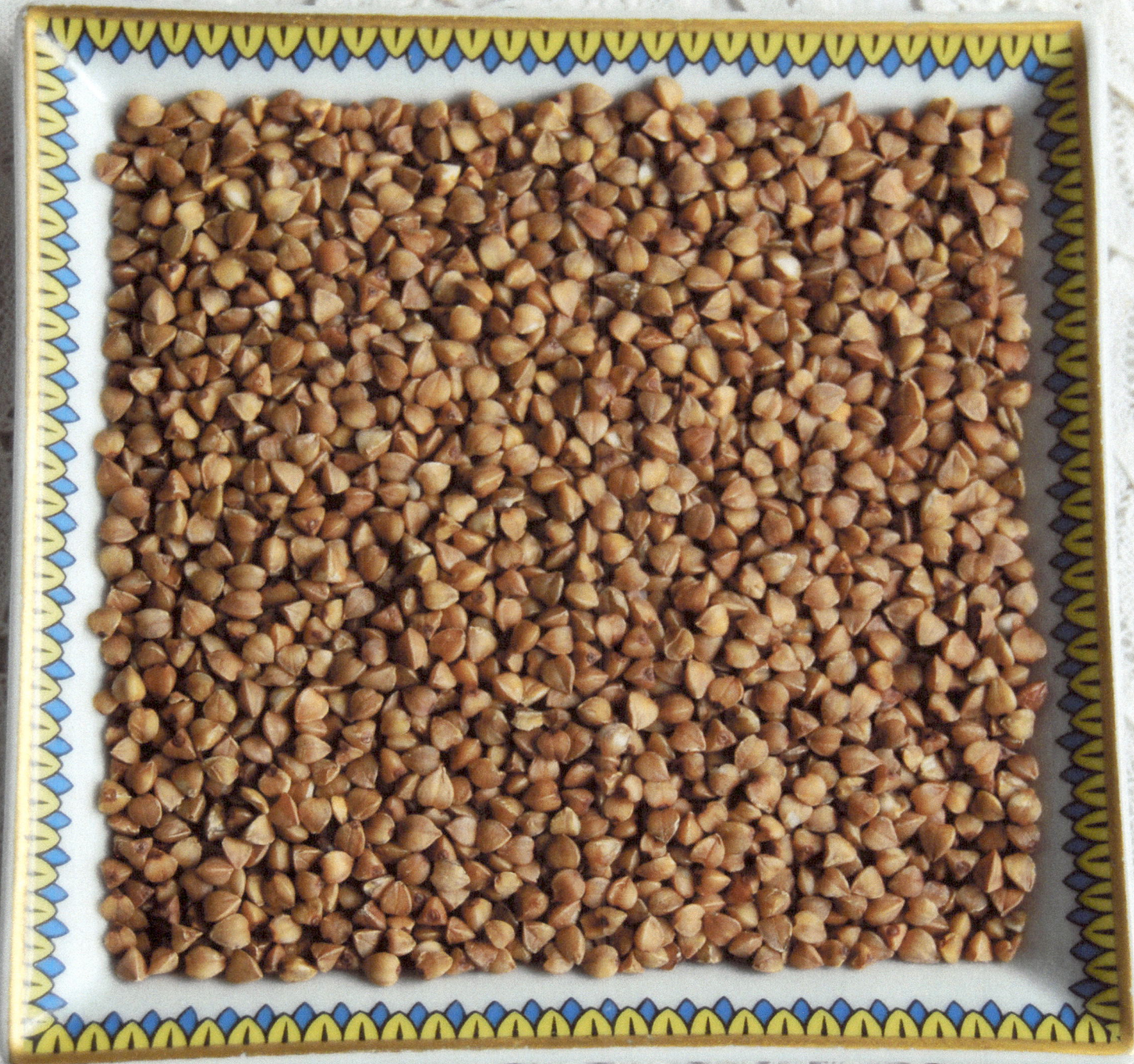

BUCKWHEAT AND BEET BROWNIES WITH DRIED PLUMS

Great way to sneak in more fiber into your dessert. Munch on these brownies on their own, with tea or coffee or take them with a small scoop of vanilla ice cream.

½ cup (125ml) boiled beets, pureed
2 eggs
¼ cup (60ml) water
1 ½ cups (375ml) buckwheat flour
½ cup (125ml) sugar
2 tsp (10ml) baking powder
¼ cup (60ml) cocoa powder
½ tsp (2.5ml) salt
1 tsp (5ml) vanilla extract
½ tsp (2.5ml) nutmeg
½ tsp (2.5ml) cardamom
½ cups (125ml) prunes chopped
¼ cup (125ml) walnuts chopped
¼ cup (60ml) vegetable oil

Makes approximately 6 squares

Preparation time: 40 minutes

In a mixing bowl, combine beet puree, eggs, water, buckwheat flour, sugar, baking powder, cocoa powder, salt, vanilla extract, nutmeg and cardamom, vegetable oil. Mix well. Carefully fold in prunes and nuts chopped up and mix again.

Preheat the oven to 180ºC (360ºF).

Take a square baking form, line with parchment paper, spoon in the batter. Bake in preheated oven for about 20-25 minutes until toothpick inserted in the middle comes out dry. Cool and remove from baking pan. Cut into squares and serve.

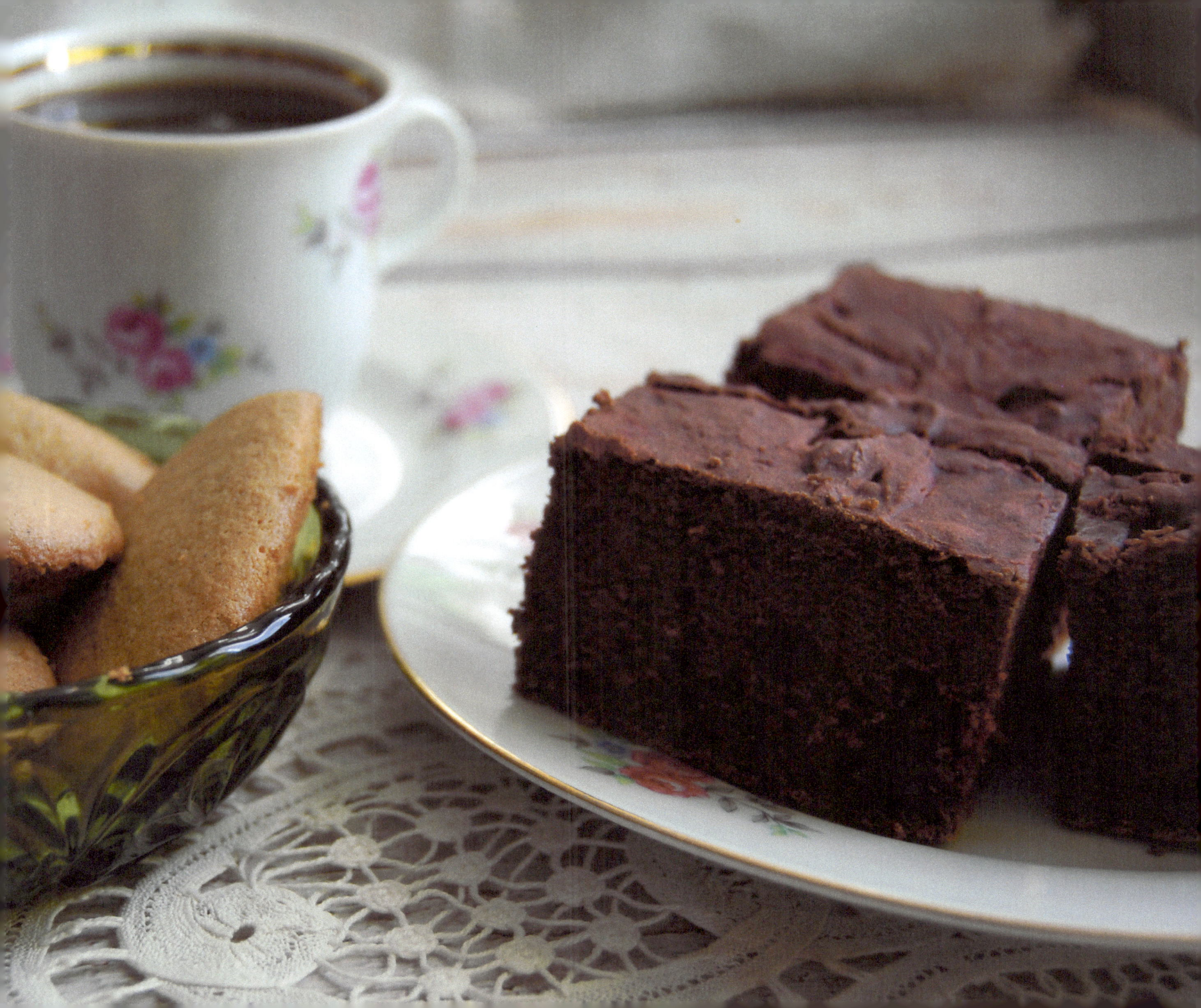

BUCKWHEAT AND KEFIR PANCAKES

Easy brunch – sweet or savoury – your choice. These
pancakes are simple and delicious.

3 eggs
1 cup (250ml) kefir, plain
⅔ cups (225ml) buckwheat flour
4 tbsp (60ml) sugar
1 tsp (5ml) salt
1 tsp (5ml) baking powder
1 tsp (5ml) french vanilla extract
Vegetable oil for frying

Kefir

Kefir is a drink made from fermented milk, somewhat similar to yoghurt. It is full of probiotics and is very helpful in maintaining healthy digestive system. Being a very opoular traditional drink in Eastern Europe it is also great in cooking and baking.

Makes 6 panckakes

Preparation time: 30 minutes

In a mixing bowl, whisk together eggs, kefir, buckwheat flour, sugar, salt, baking powder, french vanilla extract to get a smooth runny batter. You can use a blender to mix the batter too if you want. If batter is too thick, add a little bit of water (about 1 tbsp). In a large frying pan or flat crepe maker add about 1 tbsp of vegetable oil, spoon the batter into the pan and bake on medium-high heat for about 1 minute then flip over and cook another 20 seconds on the other side. Transfer pancakes into a plate and continue the process untill all batter is used up.

To keep pancakes hot untill you are done the process place the plate with ready pancakes into the oven on minimal heat.

Serve hot with apricot confiture, clotted cream, fresh berries of your choice.

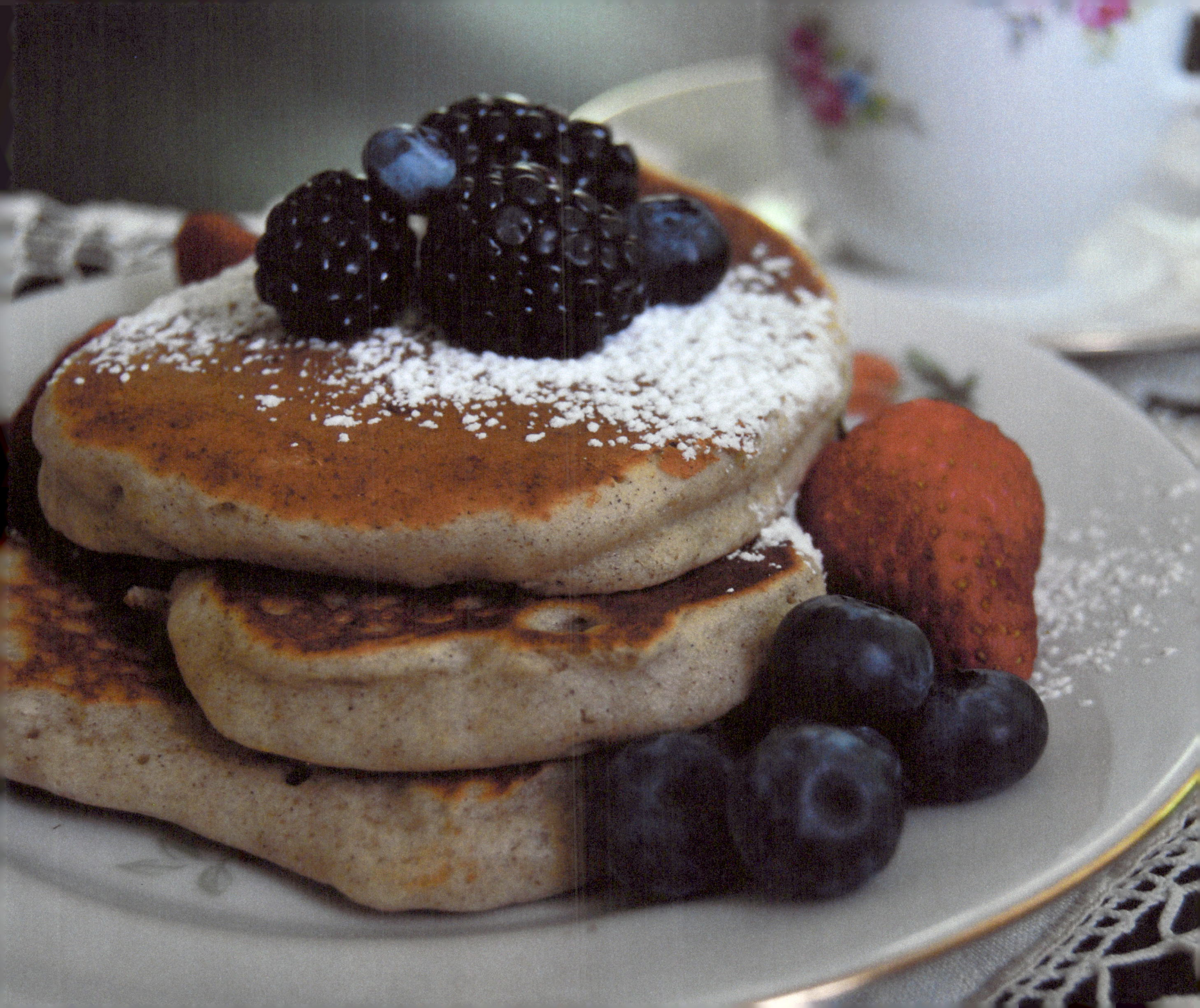

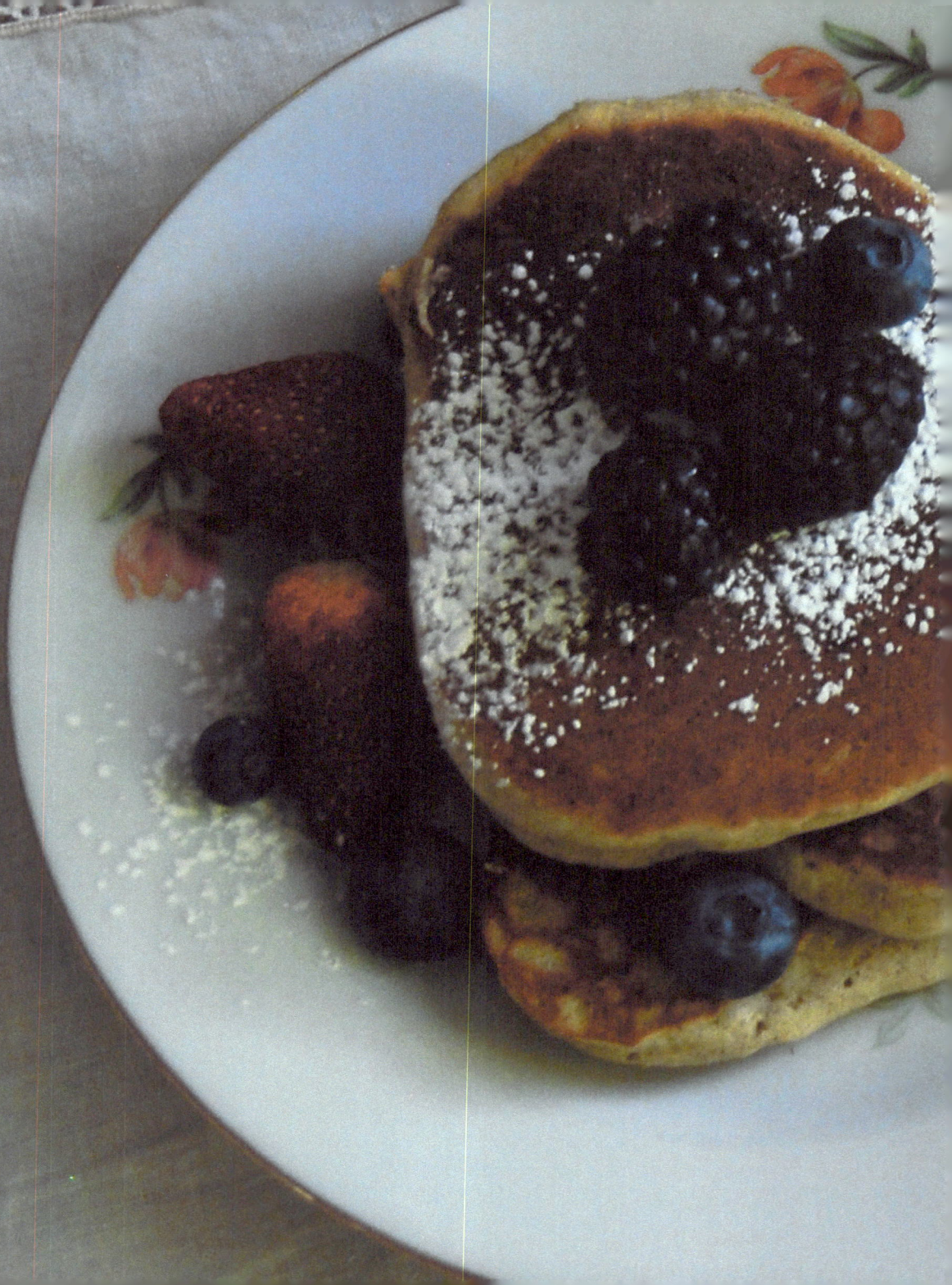

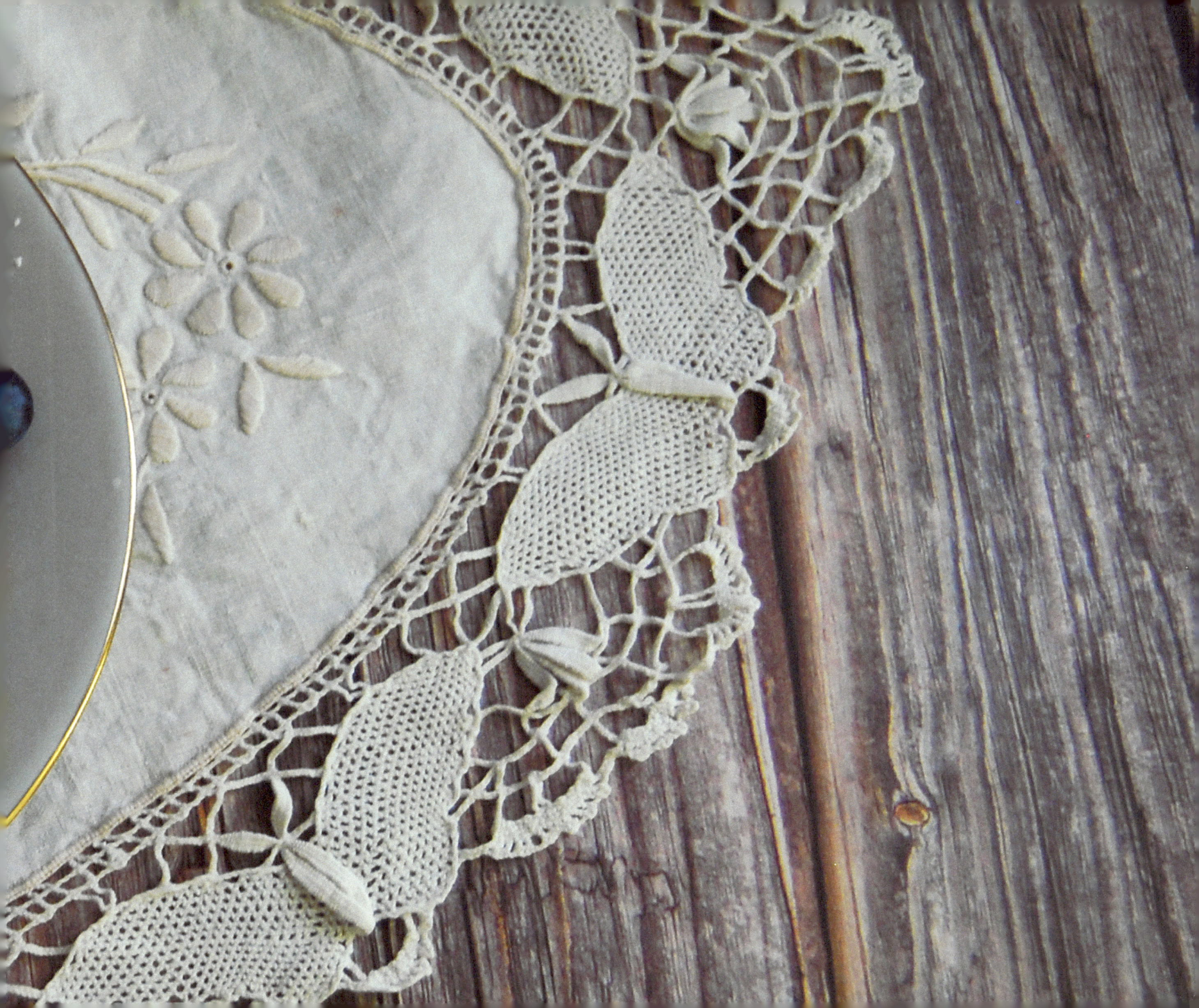

BUCKWHEAT ICE CREAM

If you do try only one recipe from this book – make sure it is this one. It is absolutely fantastic, trust me!

2 cups (500ml) whipping cream
½ cup + 2 tbsp (125ml + 30ml) brown sugar
2 tbsp (30ml) water
3 egg yolks
¼ cup (60ml) buckwheat uncooked

Pan roast the buckwheat as described on p. 31 in simple buckwheat recipe, taking extra care not to burn it.

In a small saucepan combine buckwheat and whipping cream and cook for about 5 minutes then turn off heat, close lid and let stand for about 20 minutes until cooled down. It should soften up and give off its roasted flavour into the cream. Refrigerate until fully chilled (can do it overnight).

Whisk together egg yolks. In a small saucepan, dissolve sugar in water to create simple syrup. Cool it down a bit then whisk gradually into the egg yolks – the mixture will start to foam a bit and increase in volume. Mix well and refrigerate for about 30 minutes until fully chilled.

Remove saucepan with buckwheat and cream from the refrigerator. Drain off cream into a bowl and remove all buckwheat grains. Whip up the cream into stiff peaks. Carefully fold in whipped cream into cold egg yolk mixture. Transfer buckwheat ice cream mix into a freezable container and place in freezer. Stir the mixture well every 1 – 1 ½ hours with a spatula or mixer until it sets.

Scoop out the ice cream and serve chilled. Garnish with fresh mint leaves and fresh berries.

Makes about 4 servings

Preparation: 4 hours

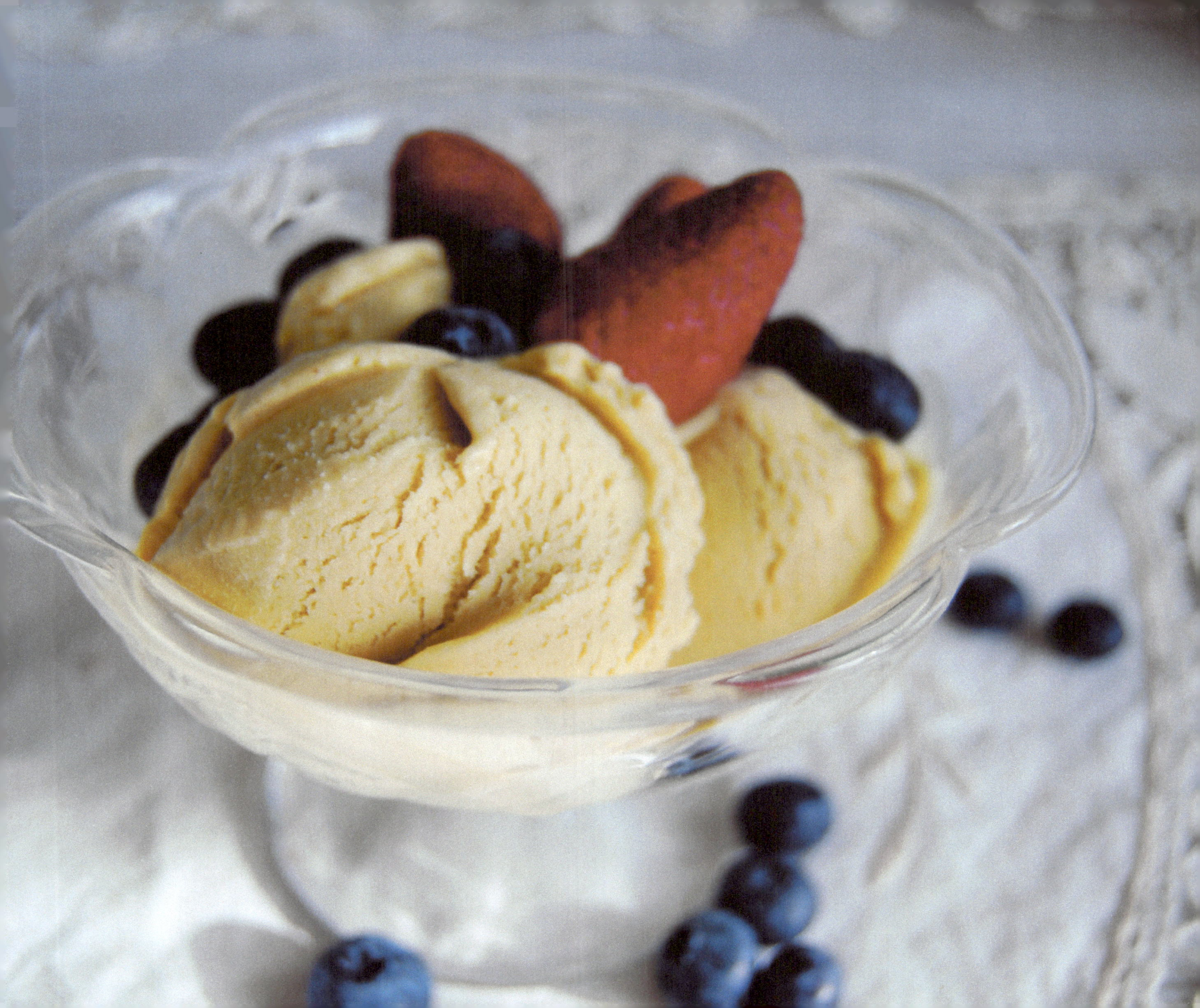

BUCKWHEAT MADELEINES
WITH MAPLE SYRUP

Kids love them. Love them so much that madeleines did not even have
enough time to cool down before they were all gone.

2 eggs
¼ cup (60ml) sugar
1 tbsp (15ml) maple syrup
⅓ + ¼ cup (75ml +60ml) buckwheat flour
1 tsp (5ml) baking powder
¼ cup (60ml) butter melted
1 tsp (5ml) french vanilla extract

Makes 16 madeleines

Preparation time: 20 minutes

Preheat the oven to 180ºC (360ºF). In a mixing bowl, whisk together eggs, add sugar, maple syrup and whisk vigorously. Add gradually buckwheat flour, baking powder, melted butter. Pour the batter into madeleine forms and bake them for about 15 minutes.

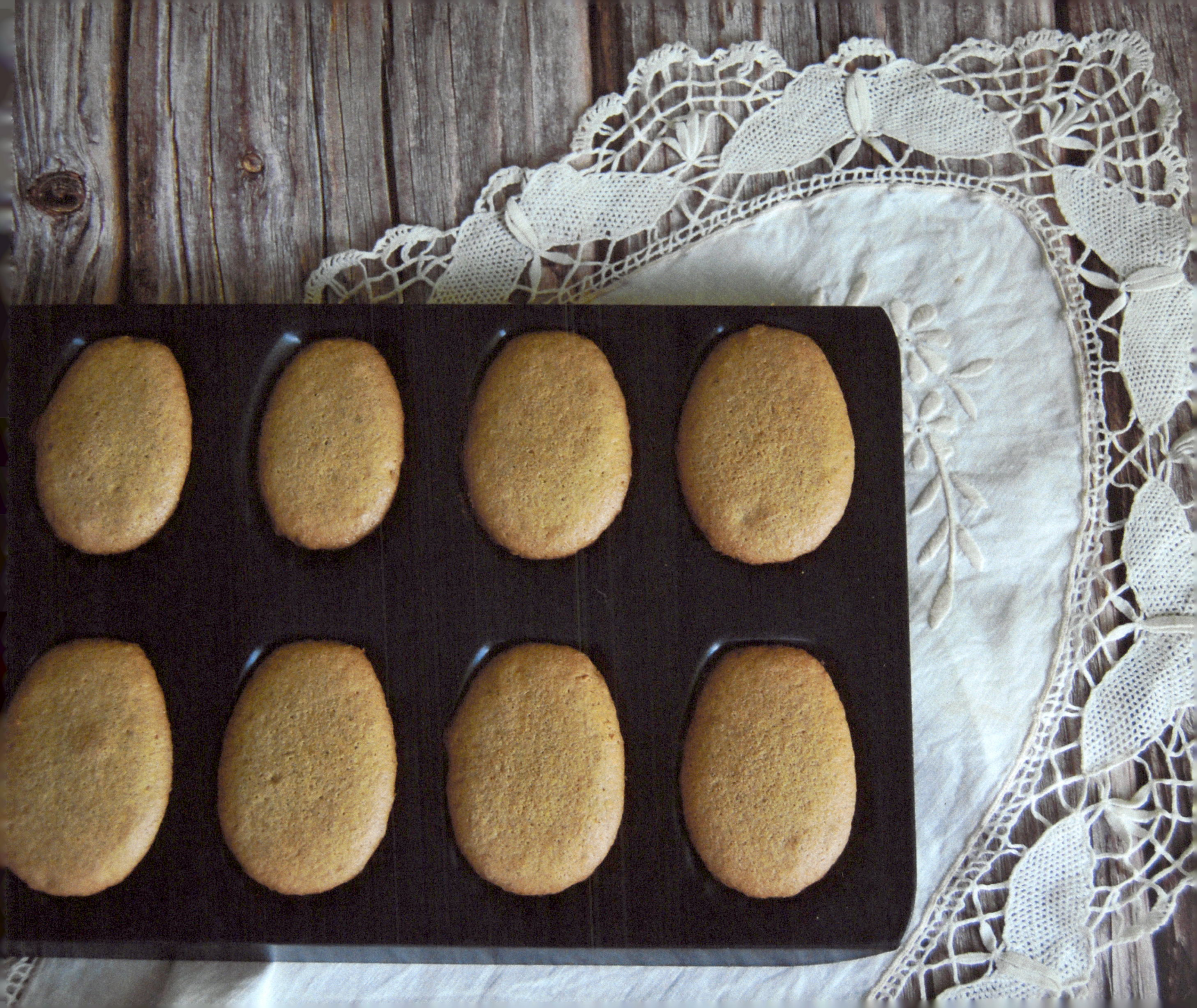

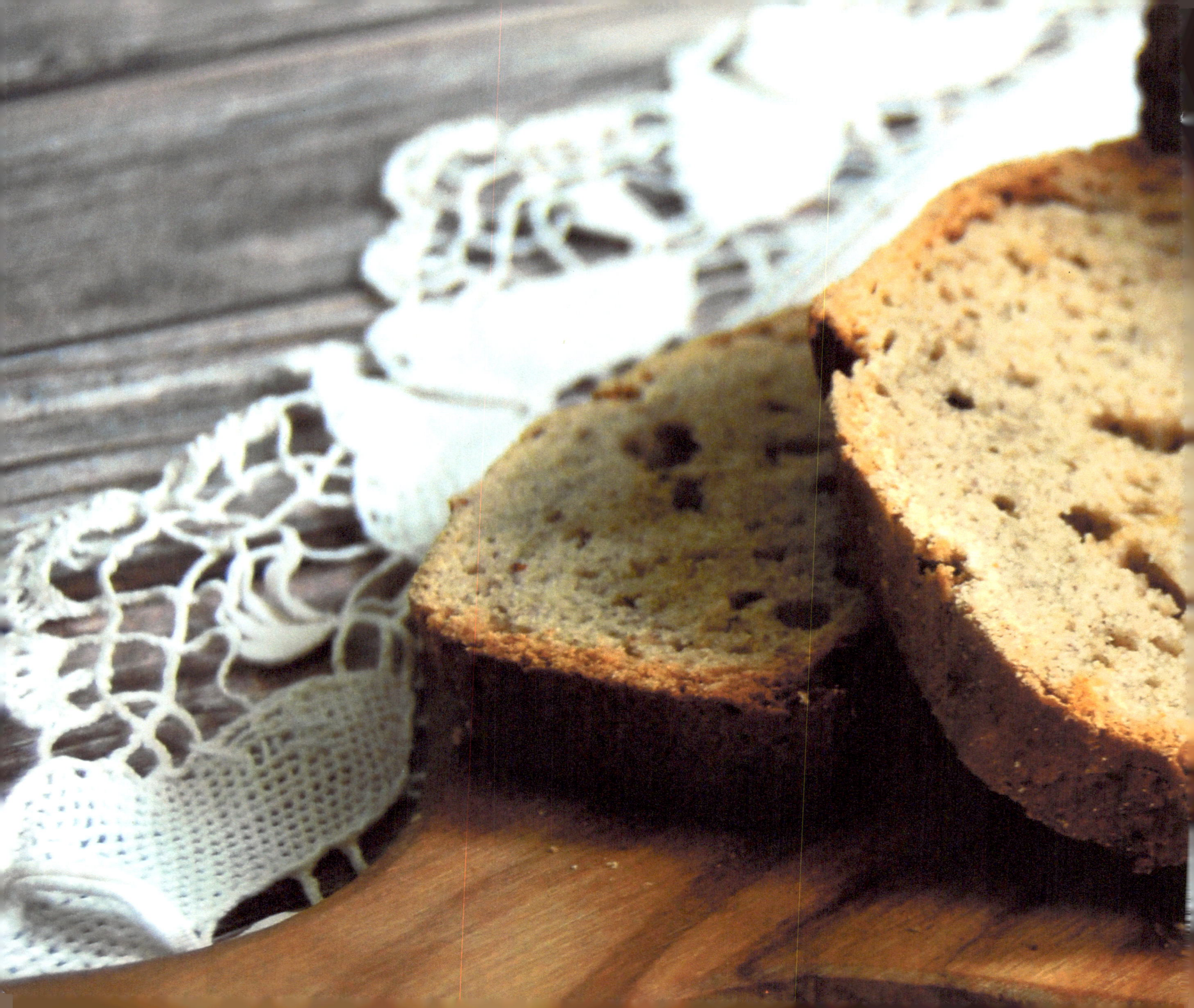

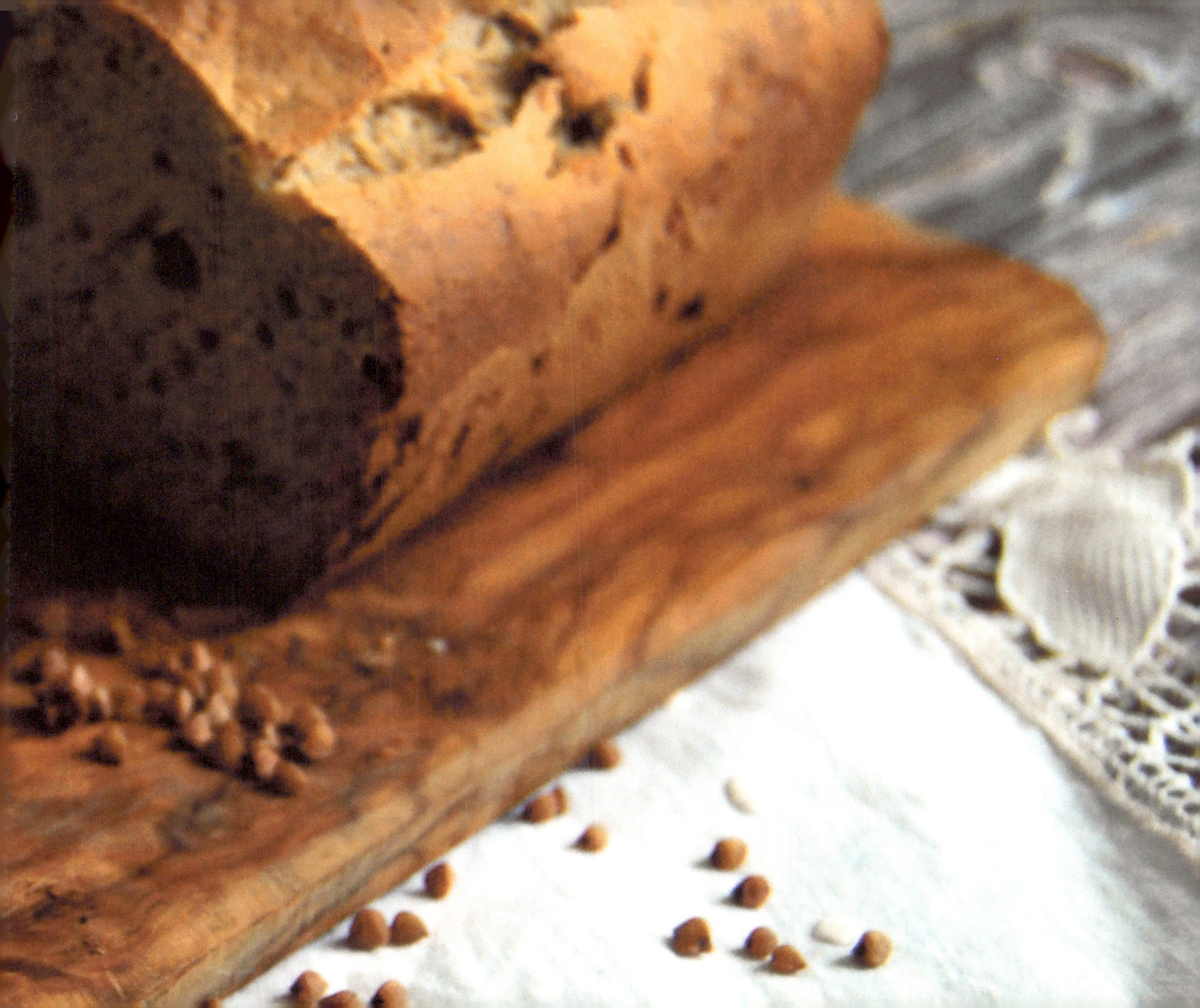

BLUEBERRY BUCKWHEAT ALMOND TART

Blueberries give a bold splash of colour and delicate flavour to this tart.

2 cups (500ml) buckwheat flour
½ cup (125ml) wheat all purpose flour
1 tbsp (15ml) sugar
1 tsp (5ml) salt
1 cup (250ml) cold unsalted butter, cubed
5-6 tbsp (75-90 ml) ice cold water
2 cups (500ml) fresh blueberries
¼ cup (60ml) almond flour
½ tsp (5ml) almond extract
1 egg
⅓ cup (75ml) sugar

To prepare the dough in a mixing bowl, knead together by hand cold butter, salt, and buckwheat flour. Gradually add about a ¼ cup of cold water to get a dough soft enough to be formed into a ball. Cover with clean kitchen towel and let rest for 30 minutes in the refrigerator.

Preheat the oven to 200ºC (400ºF). Grease tart baking form. Place dough ball between 2 sheets of parchment paper and roll dough out into a circle. Line the tart form with the dough, pierce the bottom with a fork in a few places. Place a sheet of parchment paper that was used for rolling out the dough on the bottom of the form, on top of the dough and fill the tart shell with dry beans. This will ensure the bottom is even and without bubbles. Bake the crust for 15 minutes then remove it from the oven and adjust the heat to 180ºC (360ºF).

To prepare the filling in a mixing bowl combine almond flour, egg, almond extract, sugar and mix together until smooth texture is achieved. Carefully fold in fresh blueberries.

Discard the beans and parchment paper from the tart shell and fill it with the blueberry almond mixture. Return to the oven to cook for another 25-30 minutes.

Let the tart cool down completely before removing it from the baking mould.

Makes 1 tart

Preparation time: 1 hour

BUCKWHEAT BANANA LOAF

Fantastic aroma, wonderful flavour, this loaf will be gone in a blink of an eye.

2-3 ripe bananas, mashed
2 eggs
⅓ cup (75ml) sugar
2 tbsp (30ml) oil
1 tsp (5ml) French vanilla extract
1 cup (250ml) wheat flour
1 cup (250ml) buckwheat flour
2 tsp (10ml) baking powder
1 tsp (5ml) salt
½ tsp (2.5ml) nutmeg
½ tsp (2.5ml) cinnamon

Makes 1 loaf

Preparation time: 1 hour

Preheat oven to 180ºC (360ºF).

In a mixing bowl, whisk together eggs, sugar, oil and vanilla extract. Add the wheat and buckwheat flour, baking powder, salt, nutmeg, cinnamon and stir everything together to obtain smooth batter. Stir in mashed bananas.

Pour the batter into loaf pan and bake for about 45-50 minutes until toothpick inserted in middle comes out clean.

GALETTES BRETONNES
WITH APPLE CALVADOS FILLING

This is a classic of traditional French cuisine of the Britany region. These crepes can be filled with savory as well as sweet fillings and are super easy to make.

4 dessert apples
¼ cup (60ml) Calvados
2 cups (500ml) buckwheat flour
4 eggs
½ tsp (2.5ml) salt
Water
2 tbsp (30ml) salted butter of high quality
4 tbsp (60ml) sugar

Peel and slice or dice the apples, place them into a ceramic dish and drizzle with calvados. Let rest on the counter while you prepare the galettes.

In a mixing bowl combine buckwheat flour, eggs, salt and mix well making sure there are no lumps. Gradually add just enough water to get a thick smooth batter. Let it rest, covered with a clean tea towel for about 15-20 minutes at room temperature.

Slightly grease crepe maker or shallow frying pan. Stir the batter and add a bit of water if it thickens up too much. With a ladel spread the batter onto tilted crepe maker into a layer as thin as possible, making sure it covers evenly the entire surface. Bake at medium-high heat from one side and flip over to another. Transfer the galette into a plate and keep it warm in the oven set at minimal heat while you work on the next galette. Continue until all batter is used up.

In a frying pan, melt salted butter, add apples together with Calvados and sugar. Cook on medium-low heat stirring continuously for about 5-10 minutes until apples soften up and become lightly browned.

To serve, place hot galette on a serving plate. Spoon some apples in the middle and fold edges from 4 sides inwards, like an envelope.

This dish is best enjoyed hot with some fresh apple cider to go along with it.

Makes 4 galettes

Preparation time: 30 minutes

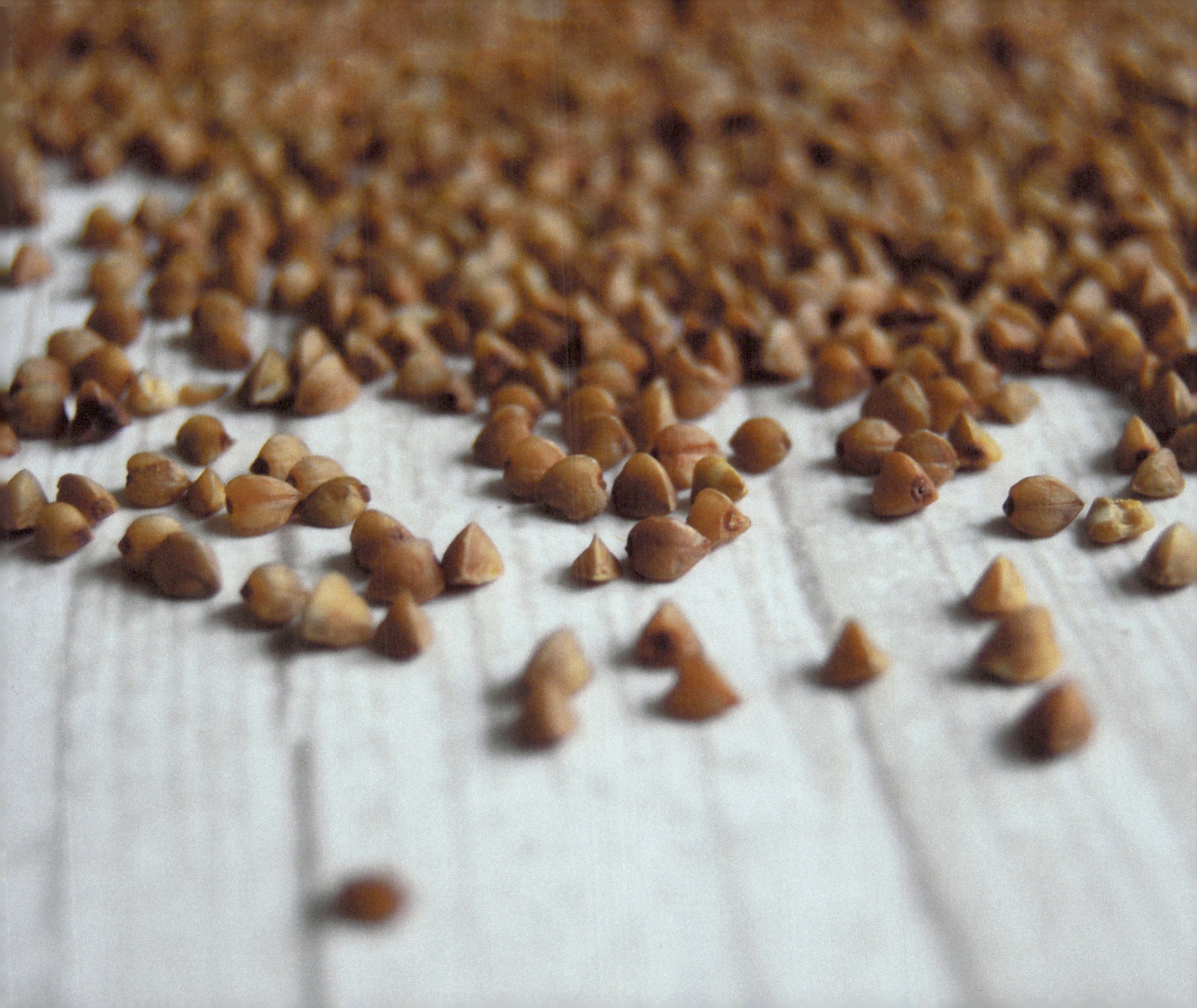

TABLE OF CONTENTS

Appetizers

Main Course

Desserts

CPSIA information can be obtained
at www.ICGtesting.com
Printed in the USA
BVHW051654170920
588989BV00002B/9